Bedtime Stories for Kids:

Magic Unicorns, Dinosaurs, Princess, Kings, Fairies, Creatures to Help Children & Toddlers Fall Asleep Fast at Night's with Positive Affirmations to Reduce Anxiety

© **Copyright 2019 by Charles Jacob - All rights reserved.**

The content contained within this book may not be reproduced, duplicated or transmitted without direct written permission from the author or the publisher.

Under no circumstances will any blame or legal responsibility be held against the publisher, or author, for any damages, reparation, or monetary loss due to the information contained within this book, either directly or indirectly.

Legal Notice:
This book is copyright protected. It is only for personal use. You cannot amend, distribute, sell, use, quote or paraphrase any part, or the content within this book, without the consent of the author or publisher.

Disclaimer Notice:
Please note the information contained within this document is for educational and entertainment purposes only. All effort has been executed to present accurate, up to date, reliable, complete information. No warranties of any kind are declared or implied. Readers acknowledge that the author is not engaging in the rendering of legal, financial, medical or professional advice. The content within this book has been derived from various sources. Please consult a licensed professional before attempting any techniques outlined in this book.

By reading this document, the reader agrees that under no circumstances is the author responsible for any losses, direct or indirect, that are incurred as a result of the use of information contained within this document, including, but not limited to, errors, omissions, or inaccuracies

Table of Contents

Introduction
The Fairies of Wisteria Grove
- *Veda (Fairy of Knowledge)*...................8
- *Celeste (Fairy of the Constellations)*...........18
- *Fawn (Fairy of the Clearings)*...................25
- *Astrid (Fairy of Universal Beauty)*...........38

Millie and the Moon Horse
- *Part 1: Ordinary Life*...................70
- *Part 2: Arrival of the Moon Horse*..........74
- *Part 3: The First Visit*...................80
- *Part 4: The Second Visit*...................89
- *Part 5: The Final Visit*...................101

The Prince and the Garden
- *Part 1: Princely Duties*...................113
- *Part 2: To Be a King*...................121
- *Part 3: A Gardener's Wisdom*...............128
- *Part 4: A King's Calling*...................141

The Wisdom Tree
- *Part 1: Cultivating Kindness*...................154
- *Part 2: Softening Anger*...................165
- *Part 3: Calming Anxiety*...................175

Conclusion...................187

Introduction

Welcome to Worlds Beyond, a bedtime story collection of fairies, royalty, and mystical creatures. This book is designed to provide children with calming and inspiring stories to help them go to sleep feeling at peace and wake up feeling positive. Additionally, these stories hold lessons to make children more aware of the world around them. They will learn about other cultures, self-acceptance, overcoming challenges, and cultivating kindness, anxiety and anger-management skills, etc. This book is designed to bring children into a deeper understanding of themselves and the world around them and find peace there.

In this book, you and your child will explore stories of fairies who bless the children of the world and teach them lifelong lessons in gratitude, self-acceptance, self-worth, self-love, healing from grief, embracing their gifts, and reconnecting. You will explore the story of the transition from an ordinary to extraordinary life through gaining a worldwide perspective and becoming open to all the world has to offer. You will read of generosity, wisdom, and the strength in being gentle and caring for others, as well as in breaking the expectations which have been forced upon you. Lastly, you will explore the problem-solving skills offered to children dealing with everyday battles such as bullying, choosing kindness, anger management, and calming anxiety.

These stories include important lessons in mindfulness, lifelong learning, compassion for others, and discovering deeper life purpose, all within the gentle and engaging form of children's bedtime stories. As children engage with these bedtime stories, they will have the opportunity to play into their natural curiosity, see where magic takes them, and grow a deeper sense of inner calm and joy. Children and parent's hearts and minds alike are sure to be touched by the characters and their stories in such a way that they will become more loving, kind, open minded and calm forces in the world around them.

We are so glad you and your children have chosen to join us on this journey into *Worlds Beyond*.

The Fairies of Wisteria Grove

Any person who has gazed upon the swaying branches of a Wisteria tree, in their shades of lavender, plum, and blue moon, can feel in their hearts that these are not regular trees. Wisteria trees are magic trees—like willow trees but with flowers in the most ethereal shades, dancing through the air. However, most people don't know that these trees do not just look magic—they *are* magic. For within the trunks of each Wisteria tree, you see dancing in the wind, you can be sure there is a village, and within that village are the Fairies who watch over and bless children with their gifts.

Before fairies are born, the Divine creator equips them with unique gifts. From the moment the gift is bestowed upon them, they are nourished and guided by an understanding of each skill and how these gifts manifest in the world. Throughout the first fifteen years of a fairy's life, they read books and listen to testimonies from the other fairies of how they can use their gifts to bless children. The fairies grow in a community of love and warmth, and eventually, the community pairs them with a mentor with whom to discover their gifts and how to make use of them in the world. Once a fairy has trained for fifteen years, they will experience a Coming of Age ceremony to disclose their gift to the world, and then begin to go out by night to bless the children.

Today, we will hear of five such fairies, each living in a different Wisteria village. Each brings a gift, and they have roles blessing children all over the world.

Veda (Fairy of Knowledge)

Veda opened her eyes to the aroma of Japanese cherry blossoms drifting through the thin papery material of her bedroom walls. She rubbed her dark brown eyes gently, staring up at the sun on her ceiling and thanking the Divine for giving her another day. As Veda's brain continued to come awake, she felt a spark in her heart as she remembered what day it was. Today was Veda's first day serving as an official Fairy of Knowledge. The night before, over a meal of moon milk, rice pudding, and cherry blossom wine, Veda had her Coming of Age ceremony. In this ceremony, she spoke to her village about her journey to where she was today. After years of training, education, and mentorship, Veda had come to define the gift of Knowledge and speak for how she would bring it out in the world. Throughout her years, Veda had learned that there are many types of Knowledge. She knew that one must see learning as a concept that always has room for change—the most knowledgeable people in the world can understand other people's pieces of Knowledge and never tire of asking questions.

Veda was so excited that today was her first day on the job. Finally, all of her hard work and intentionality over the past fifteen years would pay off, and she would, at long last, be able to bless the children. She lept from her bed and skipped over to her wardrobe, where she received her deep green velvet tunic. She opened her door to a pail of fresh water harvested from the morning dew, and she washed and brushed her teeth with it. After she was dressed and clean, Veda bounded down the hall for breakfast in the main corridor with her village's other fairies. As she sat at the table attempting to eat her rice pudding, Veda found that her stomach was too full of butterflies to eat much. Veda had learned that no matter what material things a person has, the gift of Knowledge has the power to give humans all the richness of being alive.

***

Veda spent the entirety of that day pacing around her room, unable to think of anything but her first assignment. She knew that at some point that afternoon, Fern, the village secretary, would come to her chambers and tell her where she would go that night to bestow the blessing of Knowledge. As Veda paced her room, she repeated the magical spells to herself over and over.

"May your knowledge unfold like the whole of eternity—a golden journey that never ends."

"May your knowledge arise from the sacred space of your heart—may it create a river of milk and honey in your veins."

"May you see the beauty of being a student."

"May you open like a flower at dawn to the limitless possibilities of the universe."

"May you know that in the pursuit of knowledge, everyone holds a piece of the puzzle."

"May you understand that in the sharing of knowledge, you can live forever."

"May knowledge be the wings to lift you into the essence of your life."

"May your knowledge serve as the flame—lighting every candle along the path to a better world."

"May your pursuit of knowledge be the gift that keeps on giving."

After several hours, Veda's pacing and spell-saying were interrupted by a gentle rap on the door. Veda could hardly control her enthusiasm as she threw it open, finding Fern standing there. Fern smiled a knowing smile—she was quite accustomed to this enthusiasm from the fairies in reaction to their blessing assignments. "Your first assignment, Veda," Fern said gently, "May it be all you have dreamt of, and may the world become better as a result."

Fern handed Veda a crisp envelope with lavender calligraphy which read "Veda, Fairy of Knowledge. Assignment #1." She could hardly contain her excitement as she broke the seal, retrieving from the envelope a piece of light pink paper made from the recycled materials gathered along the riverbeds. On the piece of paper was written:

"Veda,

There is a young girl named Ayu in a village not far from here. Ayu is an artist. In school, Ayu struggles to focus and does not receive good marks on her papers.

Her family looks down upon her, telling her that she is not smart enough to be successful in the world.

She is told that she will never advance in her education enough to get a good job. At school, she spends much of her time drawing and dreaming of the beautiful truths she wishes to capture in her artwork. In her backpack, she carries her art supplies, and each day after school, before the sun goes down, she walks beside a koi pond on her walk home. She stops to sit along the bank, looking at the reflection of her face upon the fish's bodies like an abstract painting. She retreats to the world where she is the happiest, where she is capable, wise—the world of art. She takes breaks to stare into the koi pond, asking the world when it will see her as worthwhile. Sometimes, she cries tears into the pond like raindrops from a sky as unclear as her thoughts. She pleads with the universe, asking why her family and teachers cannot see that she is wise, only in a way that goes beyond equations and grammar. She pleads with the universe for different talents, one that will be respected and will get her somewhere in life. As much as she loves her art, she has resigned herself to the idea that there is no proper knowledge involved in art and that it is a lost cause for her to pursue. It is your job, Veda, not only to show Ayu that the most profound Knowledge lies in the things that often only art can capture. And her family must also realize this truth. You will bless this girl by showing her and her loved ones that Knowledge extends far beyond what we accumulate in the classroom. Knowledge, like the water of the river, it is always changing."

Veda read the card a few times over, feeling her heartache more for Ayu each time she read it. She closed her eyes and began to pray that the blessings she bestowed on Ayu would be well-received.

***

Just after finishing dinner that night, Veda began to walk down the hallway to the door leading out of the village in the tree trunk. As she left the main corridor for her mission, she was met with words of support and encouragement, wishing her good luck. She felt her heart fluttering with anticipation as she pulled the handle of the door back and flew out into the warm evening. Veda flew through the evening sky with exhilaration, watching the colors change like a new paint palette every few minutes. The art of it all inspired her and made her think of all the Knowledge available in nature itself.

As she flew towards the village, Veda continued to rehearse the spells in her head, praying that she would know which blessings to bestow. Veda knew that Knowledge comes in every form and that art can go even beyond the power of language, teaching people and making them feel things they never have before. She wished she could tell Ayu this—that artists are perhaps some of the wisest people on the earth to make patterns math cannot solve and create feelings that language itself cannot describe.

Veda arrived at the village just as dusk was falling, and as she followed the arrows on the card which mapped her to Ayu's home, she saw a girl with two pigtails bounding up the hill. The girl wore a plum-colored backpack over her school uniform, and Veda noticed that her hands, stained with pale pink and mustard yellow paint. Veda hid in the branches of an oak tree as she watched the girl open the door to her home. Once Ayu was inside, Veda fled the branch, fluttering over to the windowsill. She peered over, watching an exchange between Ayu and a woman with tired eyes who handed her a plate of leftover dinner, which had gone cold. The woman seemed to be scolding Ayu, which Veda could tell simply by how she held her body. She watched Ayu quietly eat the food, not moving her eyes from the table. She ate quickly, trying to get to her room as soon as possible.

Veda switched her location to the windowsill just beyond Ayu's bedroom. She peered through the soft light of the bedroom to Ayu, sitting at her desk with a face creased in frustration as she tried to study the math problems for tomorrow's exam. Sometimes, Ayu shook her pencil in concentration, sometimes she wrote and then immediately erased it with bold movements, and other times, she moved her eyes from the paper and stared blankly at the wall. Veda could see the defeat in Ayu's face and the feeling that she would never amount to anything. Her eyes looked solemn with the thought that the Knowledge she had was the wrong Knowledge and that with it, no one would ever think her smart or capable. As far as Ayu knew, the kind of knowledge artists had wasn't necessary.

After several hours of wrestling with her math problems, Ayu grew too tired to continue. Before going to bed, she flipped open a journal and grabbed one of her charcoal pencils from her bag. Ayu's small hand began to glide across the paper in quick, effortless movements. She drew a girl sitting next to a koi pond, tears falling into the water like rains from a massive cloud.

***

Once Veda was sure that Ayu was asleep, she began to rub her hands together. "Let the walls of this place melt with magic. Let me transcend them with the intention of blessings." Veda rubbed her hands together and counted to five while keeping her eyes closed. When she opened them, she was inside Ayu's room, hovering just above her bed. Veda knew she did not have much time. She hovered above Ayu's silky black hair, strewn across her pillow in ebony wisps.

Veda closed her eyes, and a dream began to materialize. In Veda's dream, a young woman wore large framed glasses and wrapped a silken scarf around her hair. Her clothes hung away from her body like flowing prayer flags, and her skin was aglow with joy. The woman woke in the morning with a smile on her lips, and she went out to the garden, where she began to paint.

Before painting, the woman spoke into the garden: "Garden, what do you have to teach me today?" She closed her eyes and listened to the rustle of the wind through the wildflowers and the bubbling of the creek nearby. Suddenly, the woman knew in her heart that the lesson she would learn today was heart-opening. Her eyes found a bright pink bleeding heart flower, still sparkling with dew, and she heard its wisdom before her. "For the world to touch you, you must open your heart to it every morning. To open your heart, you must let the pain of the past fall away, leaving the petals of your heart light. Let them fall away to meet the sun; meet every person with the warmth they need to tell their story. Take their story into your heart and continue to grow, opening every morning, again and again." The woman's hand began to glide across her canvas in quick, effortless movements as she painted a bleeding heart, sparkling with due in the morning sun.

When the woman finished this painting, she gathered up her art supplies into a yellow canvas bag and set out for the market. On her way there, the woman felt her heart opening to every person she greeted, knowing that each of those people held a piece of a puzzle in understanding the world.

Finally, she reached the market, where a young boy played the violin, and vendors lined the road with their goods. The woman bought herself a pastry and rosehip tea and found a place to sit on the edge of the road. As she sat, paintbrush poised in her hand; she waited for the first passerby to approach her.

The first passerby to approach her was a man who lived on a street corner. He came to her and asked if he might have some breakfast. The woman bought him a pastry, and they began to talk. She told the man she was a painter, and he told her he used to be an astronomer.

The man asked the woman if she knew it was possible to see back in time. She could not understand this and asked him what he meant. The man told her that because light takes time to travel from one place to another, the farther you look into space, the farther back in time you see. The woman was fascinated. She did not know that astronomers could also be time travelers. The man continued to share his Knowledge about space with her, telling her how grateful he was to have another human who saw him as wise.

When their conversation finished, the woman painted a galaxy. That evening, the woman packed up her belongings and began to head back to her home. On the way, she saw four children playing on the street. She stopped to ask them about their game. The children told her, "We are searching for the fairies! They live in the grove, just over there." One of the girls was pointing across the road, to a grove of Wisteria trees darkening with the dusk. The woman looked at the children and asked them to say more about the fairies they were searching for. "You can't see them during the day, and even at night, it is hard to find them. They leave their homes in the tree trunks and go around the villages to protect children like us and bring us the gifts of joy and peace. The adults never see them, but we know that they are there. The things the adults can't see are the things that bless us the most." When the woman reached her home that night, she drew an image of a fairy, hovering over the village and sprinkling her blessings down like stars.

***

As Veda closed her eyes and saw this image, Ayu was having the same dream. When Veda opened her eyes, she rubbed her hands together again, just over Ayu's head. Veda knew in her heart exactly which spell she should say. "Ayu. May your Knowledge serve as the flame—lighting every candle along the path to a better world." The flame was Ayu's artistry, and the path to the better world was the understanding of how Knowledge extends far beyond the classroom.

The blessings of this spell sprinkled down on Ayu's cheeks like stars.

At once, Veda flew from the bedroom and through the house to the room in which Ayu's parents slept. Veda hovered above them, rubbed her hands together three times, and generated the magical spell Ayu's parents needed to see their daughter's brilliance. "May you know that in the pursuit of knowledge, everyone holds a piece of the puzzle." Suddenly, Ayu's parents began to dream of their daughter's work on display in the most prominent art museums around the world. They saw the way people's brains churned in thought as they looked at Ayu's paintings, and each of them walked away, having learned something new about the world. "This artist has seen things that our eyes alone cannot see. What brilliance she has. How much wiser we are to have seen her work."

That night, something stirred in the hearts of Ayu and her parents. Even in sleep, they smiled. At last, they became aware of the flame in Ayu's artistry and how it made her see the world. Her passion for art was enough to set the world on fire; to shine a light on the things many people's eyes can't see.

Veda felt a sense of rest in her heart as she knew she had finished her work. She began her flight back through the night towards her Wisteria tree, amazed that she had also grown in wisdom from blessing others.

***

Celeste (Fairy of the Constellations)

In Celeste's fairy village, no one was born to parents. They all appeared to the village on the wind in seedpods gathered by the other fairies and brought inside. The fairies sang songs and nourished them until the baby fairies inside felt safe to emerge into this new space. It took the village's entirety to raise the fairies, tend to them, and help them understand their gifts. Death in the fairy village did not look quite the same as death in the human world. When a fairy reached the end of their mission of blessing in the world, the light in them went out, and their bodies reduced to golden dust. This dust was then scattered far and wide, taking on new forms all across the universe.

Celeste knew a lot about such processes because her gift was understanding of the Constellations. Because of this, Celeste knew things other people didn't know about the cosmos. For example, she knew that when stars die, they recycle themselves into human beings, and when human beings die, they return to heaven as stars. The most important part of this to Celeste was the fact that when someone passes away, they are not gone. They live on as a soul of the galaxy, dancing in the ecstasy of eternity and watching over those who are still on earth. Heaven is the place where the dust from all the stars swirls in an everlasting dance.

Sometimes, it reconfigures into new human beings on earth, and sometimes, it watches over them. No matter what, there is a sense of unity among every star, and every human being, and dying is only the process of one becoming the other.

Celeste was most often sent on missions to bless the children whose loved ones had become stars.

Even though it is beautiful how stars and human beings are all the same, it feels sad and lonely to lose the ones we love most on earth. Celeste's job as the Fairy of the Constellations was essential because her blessings made children on earth who felt lost and alone feel whole again.

Celeste's work took great energy of the heart to complete, and therefore, she could only do it when the moon was full each month. On every other day of the moon cycle, Celeste had to work to restore her energy. She took walks, wrote poems, and bathed beneath the sun, moon, and stars, letting their messages soak into her skin and make her stronger for her work.

Every month, towards the end of another moon cycle, Celeste laid in the grass beneath the moon, breathing in the coolness of the night. Her eyes glided from one star to another, feeling embraced by all of them, as if she too were joined in their cosmic dance. She closed her eyes and began to pray for the strength she needed in this next period of the full moon to bless all the children who had lost someone and show them that they were not alone.

***

On this particular month, Celeste was following her recharging routine just as she always did. She glanced up at the moon and saw its face was three-quarters white and shining. She could not help but smile and breathe it in, glancing at the billions of stars sprinkled across the blue velvet of the night sky. She took deep breaths and began to recite her prayers.

"Let me be the voice who speaks to souls, telling them that we are not alone."

"Let me comfort the grieving hearts, reminding them that we all come from the same dust, and our dust will dance together for eternity."

"Let me speak to those whose love has been cut short by grief. Let me tell them that now, the love they share with those who are lost can cover an even longer distance—from earth to the heavens and back again."

"Let me be the strength for the children who hurt. Let me give them what they need to heal."

"Let me draw the maps to show grieving hearts the way home."

***

The following morning, Celeste awoke late. Her energy had needed longer to replenish, as the journey of soothing grieving hearts is not an easy one. She slid out of bed and saw beneath her door an envelope with lavender calligraphy. Celeste took a deep breath as she broke the seal and retrieved her assignment.

"Celeste,

Monte and Sylvia are two children who have lost their father. His body and voice have passed away, and the children cry for him every night and day. When they do not cry, they feel even worse, for all they feel is the emptiness left by their father. They do not know where their fatherly love can go now that he is gone, and they mourn every moment of their earthly lives that he will not be there in physical presence.

Their hurts feel hopeless, and they cannot understand. You are called to seek out their father's star in the sky. It will be the first star you see after dusk falls tonight, and it will grow to shine the brightest of them all. After you have found it, you must go to the children. Soothe their hearts and bless them with the Knowledge of the place in the sky where their father looks down upon them. Help them know that the first star in the sky that meets their eyes each night is their father, shining upon them with protection, guidance, and unexplainable love. When they look up at this star, let them know that they are never alone and that one day, their dust will dance in heaven with their father."

Celeste continued to rest throughout the day, preparing herself for this mission. She waited until just before dusk to set out on her mission, leaving the trunk of her Wisteria village and entering the outside world, where pain and loss and were familiar. She laid down in the grass and prayed for her eyes to be vigilant and quickly find the star, which was Monte and Sylvia's father. Her eyes scanned the sky as it changed from light blue to scarlet and rose pink, to lavender, then slate and cobalt.

Suddenly, she saw it, the twinkle of the first star. Celeste felt it warm her face and fill her heart, and she immediately began her flight. On this night, she would bring the children's father back in a way that they could hold in their hearts.

***

Monte and Sylvia lived in a red brick building in the apartment on the second floor. A metal railing surrounded the apartment's balcony with twisted bars going all the way around. Celeste found a perch on the cold metal, where she could see the family eating dinner together. When Celeste arrived, although it was after dark, Monte and Sylvia were alone in the house. They huddled on the couch, watching TV together, although neither of them knew what it was they were watching. A few minutes later, their mother bustled through the door. Her hair was messy, and her cheeks pink from the evening.

In her hands, she held a plastic bag filled with takeout Chinese food. The family had not eaten a home-cooked meal in days. Celeste watched as they sat around the TV, eyes like hollows in their cheeks, taking a few bites of their Chinese food until their stomachs began to reject it, and Monte and Sylvia's mother took it to the fridge. She returned to the living room, and the three sat there, saying nothing to one another.

It was late after some time, and Monte and Sylvia's mother told them they should try to sleep. The brother and sister knew that sleep does not come easy to the lost, but they went anyway. Since the loss of their father, Monte and Sylvia could not sleep anywhere but besides their mother, making sure that she was still there on the bed with them whenever they awoke in the night. The three quietly put on their pajamas, brushed their teeth, and retired to bed, leaving the living room still illuminated by the blue light of the television.

Once Celeste was sure they had all fallen asleep, she began to rub her hands together.

"Let the walls of this place melt with magic. Let me transcend them with the intention of blessings."

She entered the living room, which was light blue with the TV light, and still smelt of Chinese takeout. She fluttered through the house to the bedroom, where she found Monte, Sylvia, and their mother huddled on a queen-sized mattress. She could feel the heaviness of their grief as they clung to one another's bodies, trying to make sure they were all still there. She flew across the room, hovering over the three of their heads. She closed her eyes and said the prayer that she felt written on her heart: "Let me draw the maps to show grieving hearts the way home." She began to sprinkle golden dust upon the sleeping faces like blessings, which would show them the way back to their father.

Both Monte and Sylvia had a dream in which they saw their father's face. In Monte's dream, he sat beside his father on a dock, staring up at the stars as they held fishing poles dangling in the water. "Son," his father spoke, "Whenever you need to feel me, look for the first and brightest star in the sky. When you see it, you'll know I'm there with you. You don't have to feel alone or afraid, for there is nowhere you can go that I will not be with you."

In Sylvia's dream, she was on her father's shoulders, and the sun was setting over the city as he carried her home. "Sylvia," her father spoke, "I want you to oversee the sky as it fades from light blue to pink, to purple, and then to a darker blue. As it does, I want you to search for the first star in the sky." Sylvia did as her father told her, and soon, she saw it. "There," he spoke, "That star is the one that holds me. When you see it, you'll know I'm there with you. You don't have to feel alone or afraid, for there is nowhere you can go that I will not be with you."

As the dust of the dreams fell upon the sleeping faces, their hearts relaxed, and they felt, for the first time since losing their father, safe. That night, Monte and Sylvia slept with the assuredness that comes to the Wayfinder, who knows how to read the stars. If you know which star to follow and hear it speak to you, you will never be alone. Most importantly, you will always find your way back home.

***

Fawn (Fairy of the Clearings)

As a fairy who was born with the gift of seeing things clearly, it was difficult for Fawn to understand why it was so hard for people to see the world as it was. She felt as though many of her fellow fairies, as well as the humans beyond her village, had veils of fog over their eyes like the kind that blankets the road at dawn. A virtue Fawn had come to adopt over her years of training was patience. Patience was essential to maintain as Fawn reminded herself that everyone sees things differently. Sometimes, people need a gentle reminder to provide perspective and make them feel more grateful and understanding.

When she was not out giving blessings of clarity to human children, Fawn refreshed herself in the clearing beyond the village. It could be risky for the fairies to go out during the day, which is why most of their work occurred at night after the sun had gone down. But Fawn needed the sunshine on her freckled cheeks and the warmth of the golden grass blades against her bare shoulders. She needed to feel her body against the ground to feel energized and have the mental clarity she needed so badly to bless the children. So, every morning, Fawn wandered out of the village right after breakfast and found her spot in a clearing nearby.

The clearing floor smelt of fresh earth and was decorated with wildflowers of so many names; Fawn could not begin to hear them all. The sun in the clear blue sky made ripples of gold on the leaves above, parting so that Fawn's body could be warmed and re-energized. She breathed in the smell of the earth around her, and the sound of the bubbling brook nearby soothed her soul. It was rare that any human came along while Fawn was at this spot—humans seemed to spend much of their lives in confined places. But whenever a human did stumble by, Fawn hid behind a wildflower or whatever sort of clearing weed or branch she could find.

On this particular day, Fawn laid next to a wildflower, which looked a lot like a daisy. She turned her face to the sun and closed her eyes, smiling softly. Her body sank into the earth, and she felt the energy of the world around her seep into her body and begin to coarse through her veins. Immediately, her mind went blank of any worries, and she could feel only bliss. She spoke aloud, praying a prayer of gratitude for the warmth of the sun and the earth that lived and breathed around her. What a gift it was to simply be alive.

***

Fawn laid in the clearing among the parted trees, warm sun, dancing wildflowers, and bubbling brook, until she felt the warmth of the afternoon fade into a coolness that let her know it was time to head back to the village for dinner. She fluttered away, in awe of everything that surrounded her on the flight back to her village Wisteria tree.

Once inside, she joined three other fairies at the table: Priscilla, Fairy of the Rain, Adare, Fairy of the Sea, and Leah, Fairy of the Trees. For a dinner of acorn soup, gooseberry pie, and freshly gathered dew-water. The other fairies began to lift their spoons to eat, but Fawn stuck a gentle hand out in front of her "Wait, wait," she spoke, her tone soft and yet commanding. "We should take a moment to express thanks, first."

With a knowing smile, each of the three fairies set down their spoons. "Okay, Fawn. You go first," spoke Priscilla. Fawn grinned. "I am grateful for another day under this sun," she said. Priscilla went next. "I am grateful for fresh chances," she said. Adare smiled, her eyes looking far away as if thinking back on something "I'm grateful for human touch— the way we touch one another just as the waves touch the beach." Leah went last. "I am grateful for the wisdom," she spoke. After the four fairies had expressed their gratitude, they noticed a warmth coming up from within them. It was a full warmth, the kind that made their dinner of acorn soup, gooseberry pie, and freshly gathered dewdrop water go down even better.

A few moments later, their dinner was interrupted by a frantic messenger fairy, rushing to their table at high speed. "Oh, Fawn, thank goodness I found you," she spoke breathlessly. "I've just gotten word of a family of three girls who has lost sight of the beauties of life. They need a blessing of clarity. I didn't get you an envelope today because the news has just come, but it is fairly urgent. For any day that is not met with gratitude is a day lived to less than it could have been." Fawn nodded, "Of course, I'll go!" she said. She knew what the messenger fairy said was right. An ungrateful soul was the saddest of them all.

***

After dinner, Fawn set out on her journey. As she flew, she tried to process all of the information the messenger fairy had given her over dinner. The three girls lived in a large house on Lake Arbor, just outside the city. Each morning, they took the bus into the city to attend the best school in the town. In the afternoons, they participated in most interest activities until dinner, which was generally prepared by Bruna, the housemaid. Each of the three sisters had different passions. The oldest, Morgan, loved sailing. Each day when she got home from school, Morgan changed into a linen shirt, crisp shorts, and a visor to shield her eyes from the sun. She spent several hours on the sunlit water, learning how to navigate her sailboat.

Maggie was the middle daughter, and she loved to sing. Each day when Maggie got home from school, she met her vocal coach, Gertrude, in the parlor of the house. Gertrude knew how to play the piano, and she led Maggie from warmups into the rehearsal of whichever piece they happened to be doing. There, the two would stay for the next two hours, running the part over and over again until Maggie nearly had it entirely.

Maya was the dancer out of the three girls. Instead of coming home as her sisters did after school, Maya went to the city's dance studio. At this studio, Maya took ballet, pointe, tap, jazz, hip-hop, and contemporary dance. On some nights, Maya did not get home early enough to eat dinner with the family, and Bruna would leave a plate for her warming in the oven.

From what the messenger told Fawn, it seemed that the girls were blessed with an abundance of things.

Not only had they never been hungry, but they ate only the most delicious and nutritious meals as prepared by Bruna. They each had their own rooms in a large, always clean house. Inside those rooms were comfortable beds with custom bedding, full bookshelves, and even fuller walk-in closets. Bruna tidied up after them, and none of them had ever done the dishes, washed or folded their laundry, or any other such chore. They were allowed to attend the best school in the city, and if they ever struggled, their parents immediately found university professors to tutor them on the weekends. They lived in a beautiful place where they could spend endless days on the lake swimming in the summer, boating in the fall and spring, and ice skating in the winter. The girls were met every Christmas and birthday by piles of presents, always the newest thing, and never an item on their list left out. Each year, Morgan, Maggie, and Maya's parents planned a trip to visit a new place. Their parents valued travel, and they went on at least three vacations per year. It seemed that not only did the girls have plenty in their life, but they also had more than many.

Despite having all they had, the messenger fairy told Fawn that they could not find any beauty in their lives. On that day, in particular, Morgan had picked a fight with her mother about the fact that she *still* did not have the new sneakers she had asked for last week and that she was falling behind the other girls at school. Maggie came home and griped about her singing lesson, saying she was bored and would much rather lay about and not have to do anything.

Maya had thrown a fit that morning and missed breakfast because she couldn't find a lipstick that perfectly matched her strawberry shirt. Once she had searched through all of her lipsticks, she threw one across the room in anger. She could not feel entirely pretty without it. Later that day, she showed her mother pictures of the one that perfectly matched her strawberry shirt and demanded it is ordered for her immediately. That night at dinner, Morgan and Maggie spent the entire time on their cellphones, refusing to speak with one another or their parents. They got up from the table and said nothing to Bruna as she came to clear their dishes away. When Maya got home that night, she complained of what there was to eat, asking her mother, "Why can't Bruna remember, I don't like to have my pesto with *so much* basil?"

When Fawn heard this story, she nodded patiently. While it hurt her to hear of such ingratitude, mostly because she knew of the magic that could be found in thankfulness for the gifts one has, she was accustomed to such stories as this. It was not uncommon for humans to miss all the blessings of their lives, and oddly enough, it was often the ones who had the most opportunities and physical objects that had the least gratitude. To Fawn, this was an emergency indeed. Happiness was a void that could not be filled with more money, experiences, or things but rather, with the joy at that which already exists. Many people went their entire lives doing things and buying things and never feeling genuinely joyful.

***

Suddenly, without even realizing she had passed over the city, Fawn saw a large lake spreading out in front of her. She knew she must be drawing near the home of Morgan, Maggie, and Maya. Just a few moments later, she saw it, a clean white house rising out of a perfectly trimmed lawn. The porch was expansive, with stone pillars, wicker chairs, and perfectly arranged pillows. There was a stone-encased fountain surrounded by wildflowers. Above the door was a wooden sign which read, "In this home, we love."

Fawn flew around to the back bay window, which looked straight into the living room. The house was large enough to have to switch her location several times to hear the conversations going on inside. Fawn looked over her shoulder and saw a young girl on a boat, maneuvering the sail in the evening wind as she approached the dock. Fawn flew around to another window, which looked in on a girl with blonde braids, standing enthusiastically next to a grand piano. A woman with short auburn hair and glasses was pressing madly on the ivory keys, and the girl sang, with a voice that would have been even more clear and beautiful had she been standing upright and putting emotion into her performance. The woman with the short hair stopped playing several times, saying, "More feeling, please, Maggie!" After this happened five or six times, Maggie exploded. "No, Gertrude. I'm done with this today. I'd much rather do nothing at all. I'm leaving."

Fawn watched as Maggie stormed out of the parlor and up the winding staircase to her room. Gertrude tentatively began to gather her things, preparing to leave. At that moment, Morgan came in from the lake, her cheeks pink from the cold air. "Bruna?" She yelled, "What's for dinner tonight? Please tell me it's not pasta again!" A woman with a young face and tired eyes appeared, her dark hair tied loosely on top of her head. "We have lasagna tonight, Morgan." Morgan rolled her eyes as she flopped onto the couch. "Too many carbs," she muttered.

Later that night, when Maya came home, she was also angry about the lasagna. She lifted the fork distastefully to her mouth. Suddenly, her mother appeared around the corner. "Maya!" she exclaimed, "I have something for you." As her mother wrapped her in a hug, Maya slunk away with a face of discomfort. "What is it, mom?" she asked. Her mother set a light-pink box in front of Maya on the table. She unraveled the pink ribbon and retrieved it, a lipstick tube in just the shade of her strawberry top. "Oh, thank goodness," Maya said, "I was going to die without this."

***

Fawn waited until all three girls were in bed. She was planning the dream she would give to them tonight—a dream of perspective. Once they had all drifted off to sleep, she found herself a place perched on the roof, looking out at the lights of the houses casting their reflections on the lake. She did not need to go inside for the dream she would project to the three girls, and she preferred to stay outside—the cool of the night kept her focus.

At that moment, Fawn closed her eyes, and Morgan, Maggie, and Maya began to dream. In the dream, they found themselves in the city's neighborhood, on the complete opposite side from where they went to school, and Maya attended her dance classes. They saw a building made of brown brick, with windows shielded by wire bars. From the outside, it almost looked like a prison. Three adults were sitting on the stone steps, one with a beer in his hand, one with a newspaper, and one eating her dinner.

In the dream, the girls found themselves inside the apartment building in a yellow-walled corridor that smelt of stale smoke. They went up the stairs to a room on the fourth floor and found themselves inside. There was a pot of water boiling on the stove. In the living room was a girl about Maggie's age, listening to the same album on repeat in a CD player she had found in the alleyway one day. She had a book open in her lap and was writing furiously about "Music Artists of the '70s." The girl had a smile on her face.

***

Fawn spoke to the girls in the dream. "This is Gretchen. Every day, Gretchen has to run out of school and down to the bus stop because her mother relies on her to get home and help with dinner. Some days, she stops at the grocery store with a few dollars in her pocket or at the pharmacy to pick up her mother's medication. Whenever she does, she has to wait in line for hours for a consultation to get the price where they can afford it. When she gets home, she balances her time between cooking, tidying up, and studying. She dreams of being a musician, but her mother always tells her it doesn't pay well enough, especially for the people who can't get lessons or other experience.

Gretchen dreams of joining her school's choir, but the family doesn't have the money for it, nor does Gretchen have the time. And yet, every night, she finds joy in having dinner with her family and being able to listen to her scratched CDs on the player she found in the alleyway."

A few moments later, Gretchen went to the kitchen and poured a single macaroni box into the boiling water. She stirred the pasta and once it was cooked, poured a splash of milk and a packet of cheese into the mixture. She retrieved four small bowls from a cupboard, spooning the mac and cheese between them. She took two of the bowls and began to make her way down the hallway to a bedroom on the left. Inside the bedroom was a sagging bunk bed and a futon bed. "All three sisters sleep in this room," Fawn spoke through the dream. On the futon was a girl, so small her body barely appeared through the dark blue blanket spread over her.

Gretchen tiptoed across the floorboards, heavy and creaking beneath her feet. She tapped the young girl on the shoulder, "Gracie," she whispered, "it's dinner time." The girl rolled over sleepily. Gretchen helped to prop her sister up. As Gracie's small body rose over the covers, the girls saw that she had two knobs where arms go. Her legs were short and bowed. "Gracie has a genetic condition which made her arms stop growing early, did not give her hands, and made her legs short," Fawn spoke to the girls through the dream. "Each day, it is Gretchen's job to care for her. Gracie loves to watch dancing shows on television, and she often dreams of how one day, she will learn how to dance in the body she has."

In hearing this, Maya felt her heart stir. She had never thought of how lucky it was to have a body that could easily dance. Gretchen sat in the bedroom for a while, feeding Gracie her bowl of mac n' cheese. Once she finished, she kissed her sister gently on the head and walked down the hall to another bedroom. As she opened the door, clothing and objects spilled out into the hallway. She had to push hard to wedge her body through into a dark room in which no surface of the floor could be seen. "Mama?" Gretchen called through the dark. Among the mess of covers on the bed was a woman's body. "Gretchen, hello," the woman spoke. Gretchen went over and handed her the bowl of mac n' cheese. "Thank you, darling," the woman spoke again, squeezing Gracie's hand for a brief moment.

"That is the girl's mother," Fawn explained. "She is very sick, but not the kind of sickness that sits in the body—the kind that sits in the mind. Her sickness is sadness. Every day, Gretchen has to care for both her mother and her sister Gracie. There is no time for her to be a part of the choir or anything else, but she finds music in her daily life anyway."

Suddenly, there was the noise of a key in the door. Gretchen bounded into the living room. A taller girl with a high ponytail and a black collared shirt stained by grease came into the living room. "Gabriella!" Gretchen exclaimed, running to throw her arms around her sister's body. "I made you dinner," she said, running to the kitchen to fetch the third bowl of mac n' cheese. The two girls sat on the beat-up couch, eating their dinner together and talking about their days.

"Gabriella is the oldest of the three girls, and since their mother is sick, she is the one who makes the most money to support them. Every day after school, Gabriella goes straight to Bruno's Burgers down the street to work, and every morning, she goes to work at Carole's Coffee until her first class," Fawn explained.

Gretchen turned to Gabriella. "So, Gabs, what are you feeling grateful for today?" Gabriella smiled as though she had anticipated her sister's question. "I'm grateful for the opportunity to have another day alive and healthy. I'm grateful for you, mom, and Gracie, and the fact that even when we have so little, we always have each other. I'm grateful that we have dinner tonight, and I'm grateful for a job where I can make money to support us. I'm grateful to have such a kind sister as you, who works diligently to care for Gracie and mom and never complains. I am so grateful for you, Gretchen," Gabriella said. Gretchen smiled, grabbing her sister's hand in hers. "I'm grateful for you too, Gabriella, and all you do for our family. I am so thankful that the money you make allows us all to be together, to pay for mom and Gracie's medicine, to eat, and to keep a roof over our heads. I am grateful for music and the warmth my body becomes filled with when I sing. I am grateful for the opportunity to go to school and learn, and for the love I feel within this home. I am just so grateful to exist."

Morgan, Maggie, and Maya watched as Gretchen turned up the CD player's volume, and the two sisters swung their arms over one another's shoulders. They began to sway back and forth on the couch, smiling and singing together. They closed their eyes in the living room with creaking floors and walls that smelt like smoke, with empty bowls on the table and a beat-up couch, swaying to the music of a scratchy CD, and looking as if they could never have been happier than in that moment.

Just then, the dream faded away. The morning was rising over Morgan, Maggie, and Maya's white house on the lake, sunlight filtering through each of their curtains onto clean floors and bedrooms with everything in the world inside. Each girl awoke with a face wet with tears and a heart feeling heavy with perception. The world looked clearer, somehow.

The three sisters shuffled downstairs for breakfast together. As Bruna entered the dining room to set their breakfast on the table, Morgan spoke. "Bruna, thank you for all you have done for us." Morgan and Maya chimed in, "Yes, thank you so much; this looks delicious." Bruna rose her eyebrows, clearly surprised. But then, her lips spread into a smile, and she felt her heart begin to dance.

At that moment, Maya reached out to grab Maggie's hand, who grabbed Morgan's hand.

"Girls," Maya spoke, "what are we feeling grateful for today?"

***

Astrid (Fairy of Universal Beauty)

As the bluebirds joined in a chorus of morning song, Astrid felt wakefulness begin to spread through her body. She stretched her body in every which direction on the bed, bringing herself into the moment. She opened her eyes and began to thank the day for coming and her body for getting the rest it needed for a day full of energy and blessings. She swung her legs over the side of the bed to the warm wood floor. She stretched her arms above her head, spreading her fingertips to the sky and yawning. She moved her body in a few more stretches before shuffling across the room to the bathroom. First, she filled a cup with cold water and began to drink it, bringing her body into the day with energy and refreshing it from a night of sleep.

She then splashed cold, fresh dew-water on her face, followed by a moisturizer of cocoa butter and a spritz of lilac and rose. She brushed her teeth and looked upon her dark eyes and dark curls sticking out from her head in all directions like a field of untamed wildflowers. She began to speak to her body in the mirror. "You are beautiful. You are strong. You are wise. You are kind. You are capable." This was Astrid's morning ritual.

After she finished in the bathroom, Astrid went to the closet and retrieved her emerald green velvet tunic. After putting it on, she stood in front of her full-length mirror, twirling and striking various poses. She watched the way the tunic hugged her body and the shape it took with each movement.

She smiled at her reflection and spoke out loud again, "You are beautiful." Then, she put her hands at her heart and said, "Thank you, body, for all you do for me."

Astrid enjoyed a healthy breakfast of gooseberries, sunflower oatmeal, and dandelion tea to nourish her body. She chewed each bite of food twenty times, imagining it, giving her the energy and life she needed to do the things she needed to do that day. After breakfast, Astrid went to one of the village's gathering spots, where several other fairies were gathered. She spent the next two hours leading the fairies in moving to heal, where they moved their bodies in the way that felt good to them that day. Astrid stretched, she danced, she rolled around on the floor, she reached her hands to the sky, she moved in whichever direction her body told her to. She gave love and attention to each part of her body, reminding herself over and over again, "My body is good." As the movement session ended, Astrid made sure to compliment every other fairy. She was in awe at the beauty in every single body.

***

Later that afternoon, Astrid was in her room, resting, when she heard a knock on the door. The village messenger was there with an envelope. "This is a four-part mission," the messenger said, "you'll complete it over the next four nights." Astrid opened the envelope to see who she would bring to an appreciation of their bodies.

The first child to bless was a child named Wren. Wren was born in a body that looked like a girl, and sometimes that was good, but other times, Wren wanted to look like a boy. Wren felt most comfortable in t-shirts and basketball shorts and was the best basketball player at school—never missed a three-point shot. Wren wanted to be friends with the girls but was called weird for dressing "too much like a boy" and not liking lip gloss. However, when trying to hang out with the boys, Wren was strange for not sticking with the girls. Wren didn't like princesses or lip gloss but did like the color pink, as long as it was the shade of salmon. Wren didn't like sleepovers because girl's pajamas weren't comfortable and nail polish wasn't fun, and it was more enjoyable to practice tricks on the skateboard, play basketball, or climb trees than talk about boys. Wren would rather practice tricks on the skateboard, play basketball, or climb trees than talk about girls. What did it mean to have a body that liked girl things sometimes and boy things sometimes? Did the body not know how to be good if it couldn't choose?

The second child to bless was called Nya. Nya loved to dance, and she wore glasses the color of plum skin. Nya's favorite way to wear her hair was in two puffs on the top of her head, like soft, coiled clouds, floating in a sky of dreams of being a famous poet and ballerina. The first day she wore her hair this way to ballet class, her teacher pulled her aside. "You'll need to get a flattening iron to get your hair to stay down, and maybe some hairspray to make it stick. Ballerinas don't wear their hair that way." Nya didn't know what to do. Ballet was her favorite kind of dance, but her puffs were her favorite way to wear her hair. Why should a ballerina have to become flat, to plaster herself down, to dance? If her hair was out of her face and did not block her from seeing her dreams, why did it matter how she kept it out of her face?

The third child to bless was Ian. Ian had blonde hair and eyes the color of seafoam. He loved to play the violin. Ian's heart had some problems when he was born, and it made his body smaller than the other kids at school. He was smaller than all the other boys and all the girls. On the playground, the boys would hit Ian in different places on his body to see if they could knock him down with their strength. The girls would make jokes about Ian blowing away in the wind, imagining his small body found someplace far away. Once, when a plastic bag floated across the playground on a windy day, all the kids said, "look, there's Ian!" Everyone was laughing, except for Ian himself. When Ian asked to play soccer with the others at recess, they usually told him no. One day, they decided to let him play. "Ian, you play goalie," they said. As Ian stood in the goal, his classmates decided to stop the game and just start shooting soccer balls all at one time. Ian had seven soccer balls flying at him, and he couldn't catch a single one. He was hit in many different places, and his classmates laughed and said, "See, you can't play soccer if you're small." When Ian asked Emma if she wanted to be his Valentine, she laughed and said, "Boys have to be strong," she said, "and small boys like you aren't strong."

The fourth child to bless was Bianca. Every morning when Bianca woke up, her mother gave her only half a grapefruit for breakfast. Every night at dinner, her mother watched her as she ate, telling her she shouldn't overeat. In the grocery store's checkout lines, Bianca's mother picked out magazines with women on the front whose bodies were small, shaped in just the right places, and with the same bright eyes and shiny hair. Bianca felt like her eyes were gray, and her hair was too hard to keep down compared to them. Not only that, Bianca was the tallest girl in her class. She hated being bigger than all the other girls and most of the boys.

Her mother didn't like being big either. She always tried to eat less so she might shrink, and she told Bianca to do the same. Bianca's mother seemed afraid of anything that took up space in the room. She told Bianca to eat less, and Bianca felt weak. Bianca's mother thought that women were only beautiful if their bodies were like birds. The more grapefruit halves Bianca ate, dinner plates she pushed away before she was finished, and people she moved past in grocery store aisles or hallways at school, trying to shrink her body as small as she could, the more she, too, wished to be a bird. Bianca wanted a body small and light enough that the wind could carry her, here and gone before anyone could notice.

***

Astrid felt tears, heavy like dewdrops, in her eyes. She wished in the depths of her heart that everyone could see the beauty from which they were created. She wished they could see that just as every snowflake and sunrise is different and beautiful, so is every body type. She wished they could see that simply to have a body was beautiful, and it didn't matter whether that body was big or small, boy or girl or both or neither.

It did not matter what color the skin, what texture the hair, or what shape the eyes. There was no such thing as strong bodies or weak bodies because all bodies were good bodies that were strong at something. And yet, Astrid had been at this work long enough to know that bodies are shown as everything but beautiful. The world tells children there are special ways their bodies must be to be beautiful, strong, or worthy. Astrid's job was to show them that there is no need to wait for the body to become those things because each body that exists is all those things and more. She ate dinner and fluttered out of her Wisteria tree into the city of Philadelphia, where each of the four children lived. She decided to travel in order of the list's names, going first to Wren's home.

When she arrived, she saw the shadow of a child in the dusk falling on the driveway. Wren was wearing a loose, light blue t-shirt and black basketball shorts and dribbling a basketball from one hand to another. Astrid watched in awe as the basketball sailed through the net every single time, making a "whooshing" sound as it did. Suddenly, a woman appeared at the side of the house. "Wren," she said, "it's time to come in for dinner." Wren took one last shot and solemnly walked into the house.

Astrid changed her perch to the wooden windowsill outside the kitchen. She watched as Wren took a seat at the table, picked up a fork, and began to twirl spaghetti around it. Wren did not look at any of the other three people sitting at the table—father, mother, or sister Wendy. "Wren," spoke the mother, "I've set out an outfit for you to wear to school tomorrow.

It's so pretty—it's a pink blouse and one of Wendy's old skirts. You'll look lovely in it." Wren didn't say much, eyes still glued to the spaghetti. "Is it a salmon pink shirt?" Wren asked. "Yes," sighed Wren's mother, "I made sure it was salmon pink. But you have to wear it with a skirt." "I don't want to wear a skirt, mom," Wren muttered, "my body wasn't made for skirts." "What was your body made for, then?" Wren's mother demanded, "all girl's bodies are made for skirts." "My body isn't," Wren insisted, "my body is made for playing basketball and never missing a shot. It's made for riding my skateboard and climbing trees until I can almost see beyond the whole city of Philadelphia. My body is made for bloody knees and strong hands and balance." Wren's mother sighed. "Oh, Wren. When will you learn?"

***

After dinner, Wren was excused and went straight upstairs, holding the basketball under one arm. Wren changed into a white knee-length t-shirt with a black Adidas logo sprawled across the front. Once in bed, the basketball cast a bouncing shadow on the wall as Wren tossed it up, caught it, tossed it up, and caught it again. Watching the ball go up and down, Wren wondered why there were so few ways to be a girl and so few ways to be a boy. Why was it that Wren couldn't seem to do either one, right?

Astrid waited on the windowsill until the bouncing shadow stopped, the bedside table light was turned off, and a restless sleep commenced—a sleep of dreams in which Wren could just be Wren. Once Astrid was sure Wren was sleeping, she began to rub her hands together. "Let the walls of this place melt with magic. Let me transcend them with the intention of blessings." Astrid counted to five while keeping her eyes closed. When she opened them, she was inside Wren's room, hovering just above the bed.

Astrid began to speak into Wren's dream, with words written to bless the children who didn't know if their soul and body were a match.

"There is no right way to be a girl. Girls can climb trees; girls can skateboard, girls can wear collared shirts and crisp pants, or t-shirts and basketball shorts.

"Girls don't have to wear lip gloss, pajamas from the department store girl's section, or their sister's skirts."

"Girls don't have to talk about boys."

"There is no right way to be a boy. Boys can do ballet, wear salmon pink, and have feelings. Boys can skateboard and say, "Ouch, that hurt," if they fall. Boys can ask for help.

"Boys don't have to talk about girls."

"There is no particular body that "makes" you a boy or a girl. Some boys feel like boys all the time, but like things that girls like sometimes. Some girls feel like girls all the time, but like things that boys like sometimes."

"Some children are told they are boys, but they feel like girls. Some children are told they are girls, but they feel like boys. Some children feel like a girl some days, and a boy the next."

"There is no wrong way to be a boy, or a girl, or both. Your body is good, even if it cannot choose."

After this, Astrid began to sprinkle gold dust down like stars from a vast universe—a universe of girls and boys and everyone in between. She started at Wren's feet and legs. "These feet are good. They can have toes painted or not painted. These feet and legs can run, jump, or do ballet. They can ground this body into the earth, which has space for everyone. "After the legs, Astrid moved to Wren's middle-body and sprinkled dust all over. "The soul is in this part of the body. You can feel it; it's heavy and warm. The soul is so much more than the body—it is the most special part of you, and it lasts forever. Souls are neither girls nor boys because they are so much bigger than that. There are so many ways to express the soul—through storytelling, through movement, and rest."

Then, Astrid moved up to the chest and arms. "This chest is good. It holds the heart, which is capable of love. The heart is so big and so powerful, it can love anyone—boys, girls, and everyone in between. These arms are good. They are strong, no matter how much or how little they carry. They can make things, stretch, and wave hello. The most important thing about arms is how they can hold other people close in a hug to show the love the heart feels. "After this, Astrid moved to the neck and head. "This neck is good. It surrounds the throat, which is where your voice is. Every voice is important, and every voice is good. Every voice deserves to be free-- it is the music to the stories we live. This head is good. It holds your brain, which is capable of thinking, feeling, and learning. Life is beautiful because there is something new to learn, create, and feel every day. Every brain is intelligent, and every brain is capable of changing the world."

After Astrid had finished, she watched Wren's body relax onto the bed, entering a night's sleep in which Wren's body was good just as it was, and it would remain that way for every following day—even when Wren was the only one who knew it.

***

The following night, Astrid fluttered through the city until she reached the block of Nya's apartment. As she arrived, Astrid watched a bus pull up to the stop; the second-to-last bus of the night. She watched a young girl wearing a light pink leotard, wraparound skirt, and brown boots and carrying a yellow bag skip down the bus steps, thank the driver, and bound up the concrete stairs of a light blue apartment complex. The girl had her hair in two perfect puffs, one on each side of her head. Each puff was tied with a pink silk ribbon. Astrid flew up to the window of a sixth-floor apartment as Nya took the elevator.

Astrid watched as Nya threw open the door to embrace her mother, who was still dressed in a red apron from her work at the diner. "So good to see you, my dancing girl," Nya's mother said, holding her daughter close. "So good to see you too, mama," Nya said, burying her face into her mother's chest with a look of serenity on her face. There was soulful music playing on the record player, filling the room with even more warmth than the dim yellow light and the pot of soup boiling on the stove.

Nya and her Mama began to sway, slowly at first, arms clasped around each other, and eyes closed to feel the music. Astrid watched them sway and twirl, like two angels gracing the kitchen as if it were heaven. "Nya," the mother spoke, "show me what you're learning in ballet class." Nya's eyes fluttered quickly away from her mother's and became glued to the floor. She tried to force a smile, saying softly, "Mama, we don't dance ballet to soul music." "Well, what kind of music should I find, then?" Mama demanded. "We don't have any records with ballet music," spoke Nya, not moving her eyes from the floor. "Well, we're going to have to fix that, then," Mama said. "This weekend, we'll go to the record store, and I'll buy you a record with ballet music. That way, you can practice. Practice makes perfect on the journey to your dream," Mama said, leaning down to kiss Nya on the forehead. Nya kept her eyes on the floor, and her tongue quiet. She couldn't tell Mama that she didn't know if she'd ever be able to go back to ballet class.

***

That night after a quiet dinner, Nya stood at the kitchen sink with her mother, washing the dishes from the day. Mama was busy at the diner during the day, and Nya was busy at school and then dance class, so the breakfast dishes and Mama's dishes from her lunch break didn't get done. But Mama never let them go to bed without doing the dishes. "We always have to sleep and wake up with a tidy house," Mama would say, "It's better for the mind."

The two stood side by side, Nya washing, mama drying. Mama was humming gently, wondering to herself why Nya had suddenly become so quiet.

Finally, Nya broke the silence. "Mama," she stammered, "do you know how to do a ballerina bun?" Mama stopped drying to look at her daughter. "Just like that," she said, pointing to Nya's hair.

Nya felt her eyes fall again, this time to the bits of leftover soup clinging to the sink's metal. "I mean, a real ballerina bun," she said, "you know, the slick, straight kind that stays on the back of the head and doesn't move anywhere?"

Mama was quiet for a minute. "Nya," she said, "You don't need your hair in that kind of bun to be a ballerina." "Yes, I do, mama," Nya pleaded, "Ms. Lamberti said I have to have my hair straight and stuck tight to my head to show discipline, respect, and dedication to the practice of ballet." "Oh, did she, now?" Mama questioned. "Well, it looks like I may have to have a word with Ms. Lamberti." Nya sighed and kept the rest of the words to herself. She knew that Mama didn't have the time to flatten her hair every day, wrap it into a donut shape, and spray it down. It would take hours, and besides, Mama had to work the early shift at the diner.

This meant Nya had to take the early bus to school. Even if Mama did have the time, there were things she didn't want to change about herself or her daughter to make them look the way other people expected them to look. Mama said that there was no merit in such expectations and that the world would come to see girls like her and Nya as beautiful for precisely as they were. But to Nya, the most beautiful thing in the world was to do ballet.

The two finished the dishes, and Nya remained quiet, not knowing what else to say. It seemed to her that Mama didn't like the idea of flattening her hair with an iron, wrapping it into a donut shape on the back of her head, and spraying it down like plaster that couldn't move. Defeated, Nya decided it was time to go up to her room. Maybe if she thought hard enough, she could think of a new plan for herself. Maybe if she thought hard enough, she could think of a kind of dance where the dancers showed discipline, respect, dedication, and talent, with puffs just like hers.

***

Nya closed the door to her bedroom and flopped onto her mattress. Lying on her back, she could still see the posters of ballerinas hanging on her walls. There was one of a girl on a stage in a stark white tutu and bright red lipstick. The girl stood propped up on one leg; her pale pink pointe shoe bent perfectly beneath her muscular calf. Her other leg was angled out behind her, foot turned out, no flaws in sight. She had one arm stretched gracefully across her body, the other reaching to the sky as if reaching for heaven. Her eyes looked wistfully up at the hand above her body. It was the perfect arabesque. The girl's hair was blond and plastered back into the perfect bun.

In another poster, there was a wooden ballet barre, like the ones that lined Nya's studio walls. A younger girl, around Nya's age, was in the picture. The girl wore a pale pink leotard and skirt, with a thin black cardigan laced over the top. She had one hand on the bar, and the other angled up above her head in an arch shape. Her foot was in a tendu out in front with the excellent turnout; her body folded effortlessly over the leg. Her hair was dark, the same color as Nya's, but it too was smooth, sleek, and plastered to her head.

Nya wracked her brain, waiting for something to come to her mind that would make her happier than being a ballerina. But there was nothing. Nya's dream was to be up on a stage, calf muscles protruding like sculptures, lips painted a radiant color, stage lights beaming on her face as she glanced up at her hand as if glancing at heaven. She wanted to be the light in a dark auditorium, the radiance, grace, and control of her movements, making the audience's hearts stir. Nya wanted to be a ballerina.

Astrid watched with a heavy heart as Nya stared up at the ceiling, daydreaming until she became too tired to be awake any longer. She decided to go to sleep, where she no longer had to worry that she might never be allowed to return to ballet class. In her dreams, there was always a way to return to ballet.

***

Outside the window, Astrid was coming up with a plan. She waited for Nya to fall asleep, then willed herself inside the bedroom. "Let the walls of this place melt with magic. Let me transcend them with the intention of blessings." Astrid counted to five while keeping her eyes closed. When she opened them, she was inside Nya's room, hovering just above the bed. Nya's curls were scattered across her silk pillowcase, and her face was bunched up with tension.

Astrid breathed in, closed her eyes, and in a moment, was inside Nya's dream. Astrid brought Nya into a studio, much like Ms. Lamberti's. Except, instead of Ms. Lamberti, there was another woman, with hair in two glorious puffs, tied by a pink silk ribbon.

"Nya, my prized ballerina," the woman spoke to her with a smile. The rest of the dream was full of Nya and the teacher, practicing Tandus, grand jetes, and arabesque. With every move Nya made, the teacher exclaimed, "Brilliant! Miraculous! You are a flower petal on the breeze, Darling." After the rehearsal was finished, the woman spoke to Nya. "Darling, you are more than ready for your first solo tonight. With your grace and beauty, you will transport the audience to heaven."

The next scene flashed to a red velvet curtain, drawing up from a stage. The stage was empty, casting a light into the sold-out theater. Everyone held their breath. A few moments later, out came Nya, wearing a stark white tutu, lips the color of plum skin, and two beautiful puffs. Her calves curved entirely above her pointe shoes like the most delicate sculptures. She waited, eyes down towards the ground, arms stretched up and rippling with strength. A silence fell.

The music broke through the silence, and with it, Nya began to dance, moving so gracefully across the stage it was as if she could fly. With every movement of her body, the audience could feel their hearts stir. They watched her glide across the stage in such grace and beauty that time became an illusion—no one could think of when the show would be over, only the gift they were receiving to watch it. After the final song, as Nya curtsied, the audience jumped to their feet, and the auditorium was flooded with the sounds of a standing ovation. Shouts of "Bravo, bravo" and roses were thrown upon the stage rained down on Nya like prayers, and she knew at that moment that this was what she was born to do.

After the show, Nya stood in the lobby, greeting excited audience members who thrust their programs into her hands, begging for her autograph. She had young ballerinas coming to her, asking her what tips she could give them. Suddenly, out of the corner of her eye, Nya caught a glance at Ms. Lamberti. Ms. Lamberti stood in a corner, lips drawn down into a tight frown, looks sad and empty. Her shoulders were not postured like a ballerina but hung in defeat. Nya could not help but smile to herself.

The final scene of the dream fast-forwarded many years, this time to a different studio.

This studio had light blue walls with ballerinas of all body types and hairstyles, standing in different poses.

Each dancer was like a unique sculpture in a garden. At the front of the room, Nya saw herself. She was a bit older, this time wearing long gray legwarmers and a yellow leotard, with her hair tied by two yellow silk ribbons. All at once, students began filing in. There were boys, girls, donut buns, double puffs, and leotards hugging every shape like an omen. The students took their places at the barre, staring expectantly at their teacher, who had revolutionized the world of ballet forever. "Hello, my dancing boys and girls," Nya spoke, "Let's make some magic."

As Astrid opened her eyes, she saw a smile spread across Nya's face. There was a knowing in the face—the kind of knowing that says, although the road may not be easy, she would make it there someday. Nya's body relaxed into the feeling that there is always more than one way to create art, and the ones who are brave enough to keep trying are the ones who bring everyone closer to heaven.

***

On the third night, Astrid went back outside again into another chilly Philadelphia night. "Two down, two more to go," she thought to herself. As she flew, she prayed, thinking of both Wren and Nya. It saddened Astrid how the world tried to put people's bodies into boxes, telling them which ones belonged. She prayed for Wren and Nya that no matter how hard the world wanted to keep them inside a box, they would keep breaking out, time and time again.

She flew across the town to a park of trailer houses. Inside a trailer house painted the color of eggshells, lived Ian. As she arrived, she heard the sweetness of violin music floating out an open window at the back of the trailer. Astrid sat nearby, closing her eyes and relaxing in the beauty of it. However, the music came to a screeching halt when she heard a man yelling for Ian from the kitchen. "Grab me another drink, will ya, kid?" demanded a man reclined in a beat-up armchair, who Astrid assumed must be Ian's father. Above the TV across from the man was a photo hanging in a wooden frame.

In the photo stood the man next to a beautiful woman in a light pink floral dress. Her arms were around a small boy in between them, with the same blond hair and seafoam green eyes as Ian.

"Are you gonna eat, dad?" Ian asked timidly. "Why don't you mind your own?" his father growled back. Ian retreated into the kitchen like a scared puppy and found himself a can of Spaghetti-O's in the cupboard. As he ate them, Ian worried about two things. The first was that Spaghetti-O's lacked nutritional value, which gave him little hope of getting much taller than he was. The second was that Spaghetti-O's were not the most heart-healthy thing he could be eating. Ever since his mother had died, and Ian had been in the care of his father, his medical care was not kept upon in the way it should have been. Ian's father was too busy sitting in his recliner and being angry to care about much else.

After eating his dinner alone, Ian went back to the bedroom, where he continued to play his violin. His fingers glided back and forth along the sleek back fingerboard as his bow made perfect lines and slurs up and down on the strings. Unfortunately, the music was glorious but was cut short when Ian's father growled that it was too loud. With this, Ian put away his violin with great tenderness. This violin had been given to him by the school, and he had to take excellent care of it.

***

Once the violin had been carefully put away, Ian got ready for bed. After he laid down, Astrid waited for what felt like hours. Every time she expected him to fall asleep, he blinked again, never moving his attention away from the ceiling. Circles began to form like bruised storm clouds underneath his heavy eyes, but he could not find sleep. He blinked away his tears with heavy movements, glad that no one was in his bedroom to see him cry. He felt his heart beating irregularly, as it did every night. He wanted to know someone cared for his heart in any way at all.

His eyes wandered over to the corner of the room, where his class picture was silhouetted against the wall. Even in the darkness, Ian could pick out his shape as the smallest out of all the girls and boys in his class. His little body shuddered as he imagined the children's shouts on the playground the day before at school, striking his body like hard pebbles. "You're so weak; I could just knock you over." "Hey, look, a plastic bag! That looks like Ian. Ian, do you ever feel like a plastic bag? You sure look like one!" "Ian, do you ever eat anything? It looks like you could use a cheeseburger." "Ian, what are you going to do if all the girls you find are bigger than you?" "Ian, you're too small to be a boy." "No, you can't play soccer with us. We don't want anybody on our team that could be knocked over just by the wind." "Ian, Emma doesn't like you. She says you're too small—you look like her little brother."

Ian felt his ribs begin to shake like trees in a hurricane. The tears began to rush down his face faster and faster, like large, salty waves. He felt like he could drown. He wondered why he couldn't just be the same as everyone else. In the corner of the room, Astrid saw Ian's violin and music stand, and on the wall behind it, a photo of Ian standing with his soccer team from the year before. Even these things were not enough to make Ian feel that he was enough. Ian's body shook with the sad idea that he was too small ever to do anything significant.

Astrid waited for him to fall asleep, glancing back and forth between his bed and the rising sun. There was hardly any time remaining, he had to fall asleep sometime, or she would not be able to bless him. Finally, just as the sky was beginning to turn light blue with the dawn, Astrid saw Ian's heavy eyelids fall into sleep. He had cried until his body could cry no more, and now would get only two hours of sleep before another day of the kids at school throwing stones at his body with their words.

***

Once he was finally asleep, Astrid closed her eyes and began muttering quickly: "Let the walls of this place melt with magic. Let me transcend them with the intention of blessings." Astrid counted to five while keeping her eyes closed. When she opened them, she was inside Ian's room, hovering just above the bed. All at once, Astrid began to imagine a three-scene dream to bless Ian with.

In the first scene, Ian was running down the soccer field. He was faster than everyone else on the field, zipping in and out as if he were attached to a bolt of lightning. He was so quick; no one could catch him. He dashed past the defenders on the opposite end of the field, keeping the ball at his feet with all the control in the world. The crowd was roaring on the sidelines. Ian drew back his foot and struck the ball with perfect form.

It went sailing through the air, and even though the goalie was tall, it was too strong for him to grip it. The ball made a "whooshing" sound as it sailed into the net. Ian threw his arms up into the air, his heart pounding with excitement at how far they had made it. He ran around the field in a victory pose, and when his teammates came up to him to pat him on the back or chest bump, the weight of their bodies did not even come close to knocking Ian down.

In the following dream, Ian saw what looked like an older version of himself, with thick, black-rimmed glasses over concentrated eyes the color of seafoam, and blond hair styled with gel. He was wearing a crisp black suit over a white undershirt, and he held his violin comfortably in one hand, his bow in the other. Ian was waiting in the wings of a stage behind a red velvet curtain. He began to walk, heading towards a single gleaming music stand in the center of the stage. He reached the stand, took a deep breath, positioned his violin between his shoulder and chin, and drew up the bow with grace. The curtain raised, and as his figure became visible on stage, the audience erupted into applause. A silence fell over the auditorium, broken only by the crisp sound of Ian's symphony. It floated through the room, filling the audience's hearts with a feeling more immense than anything they had ever felt before. With the sound of every perfect note, the audience cried, they smiled, they fell in love with no one in particular, and they felt as if they could fly. Ian was brilliant, a maestro, the most prominent force in that room, and across the world, in the ear of every person who beheld his orchestrated violin pieces.

In the third scene, Ian was sitting on a park bench, studying a book of music. His soccer uniform was in his backpack, but he was eating his lunch. Suddenly, he heard a voice say to him, "eating alone today?" He looked up and was met by the most beautiful mahogany eyes, shining in a sea of freckles. A girl with flowing red hair and light pink roller skates stood in front of him, smiling sweetly. Ian felt his heart begin to beat faster with the sight of her beauty and the kindness he could see in her eyes. "Yeah," he stammered, "I'm eating alone before soccer practice." "Could I join you?" the girl asked. Surprised, Ian scooted over on the bench to make room for her. She sat down close to him, so close that he could smell the scent of strawberries coming off her hair. "What are you reading?" she asked, peering over his shoulder. "Bach," he said, "I'm studying Bach. I'm a violinist." The girl's eyes lit up. "No way!" she exclaimed, "I'm a cellist!" The two spent the next hour talking fervently about their favorite types of music. At the end of their talk, the girl gave him her phone number and asked him if they could meet for lunch the next day on the same bench. Ian's heart was pounding like an orchestra crescendo. Finally, someone who saw him for all the things he was besides small. The way this girl looked at him, the way she spoke, the way she laughed with him, the way she asked him questions made him feel anything but small.

In the final scene, Ian saw himself at a table with his mother, wearing the same light pink dress she wore in the photo above the TV. They were drinking lemonade and talking about all his accomplishments. She told him how proud it made her to watch him play soccer and zip around the field like lightning and how the music he played on the violin was enough to make her feel as though she had gone to heaven.

She spoke gently, telling him that although she knew how much it hurt him to be harassed and bullied by his classmates for being small, he was anything but a small presence in the world.

She told him his persistence in overcoming his classmate's hurtful words and actions was enough to restore her faith in the power of perseverance and healing, and she was inspired by him every day. Tears streamed down his mother's face as she told him how grateful they should be for the fact that Ian's body had overcome his heart problems and kept him alive, healthy, and capable of doing so many things. With that, she reached out for his hand. "Let's say a prayer, shall we? Let's express our gratitude for the goodness of our bodies and all they have done for us." And they did.

As the dawn began to rise outside the trailer home, a smile spread across Ian's face, and his heart began to beat with new anticipation. He was worthy of love; he was not small; he would change the world—and he was grateful to his body for getting him there.

***

On the fourth night, Astrid arrived at a townhouse. A young girl sat on the steps; a yellow moleskin journal spread open in her lap. In her hand was a pen, furiously scribbling the same words line after line. "Why should I shrink? Why should I shrink? Why should I shrink?" Suddenly, a woman threw open the door. "Bianca, you were supposed to be inside thirty minutes ago. I don't want you coming to the table like that. Go take a shower; I'll save you something to eat." Knowing she would go to bed hungry, Bianca walked solemnly up the stairs with her head down.

After Bianca finished her shower and came to the table, her two brothers and father ate chocolate cake. "Not for us, B," her mother said, setting a plate of spinach and half a chicken breast in front of her." As Bianca chewed her food, she could feel her mother's watching her like a hawk. She felt her mother's eyes on each part of her body, willing it to be smaller. As her mother willed this upon Bianca, her discontentment deepened like a hole in the earth. Bianca felt like her mother would soon be swallowed up.

When Bianca's mother tired of watching her eat, she picked up the magazine she had grabbed in the grocery checkout that afternoon. The woman on the front had glowing golden skin, clad by a bubblegum pink bikini that rose from the flatness in just the right places. Her smile was broad and glimmered like fresh snow under the afternoon sun. Her blonde hair cascaded down her back like a waterfall of silk and her eyes were the color of the ocean—sparkling as if they had never seen anything that hurt. Most importantly, though, this woman was small in every way she was supposed to be. She took up only the amount of space she was supposed to take up. Bianca watched her mother shift uncomfortably as she flipped through the magazine, looking down at her belly, her thighs, her own feet, and wishing she could fade away from them.

***

That night as she laid in bed, Bianca could not fall asleep. She tossed and turned, feeling the pain of never being good enough. Why was her mother so afraid of bodies taking up space? Bianca closed her eyes and began to scan her body. She was eleven, which meant she was only going to get bigger in her mother's words.

According to everything Bianca was being told about bodies, that wasn't a good thing. With her eyes squeezed shut, Bianca began to bring attention to her feet at the end of the better. She began to squeeze the muscles in her feet as hard as she could, saying to herself, "Please, stop growing. Please, stop growing." As she did, she imagined never having to buy shoes that were at least double the other girls' size. She imagined never having another person tell her she had such big feet.

Next, Bianca moved her scan to her legs. She was only eleven, but she saw the way her mother stared at her thighs, which were becoming more like tree trunks every day. Bianca had always looked upon her mother's thighs and felt that there was power there, but according to her mother, it was best to strive for a gap between thighs through which the sun could shine. "Please, don't let my legs become thick like tree trunks. Let them be small and weak; instead," Bianca spoke to no one in particular.

The next place Bianca moved her attention was to her hips. Her mother had hips so expansive, Bianca imagined they could carry enough love and nourishment for the entire world. Bianca had always loved to watch her mother on the rare nights that she gathered with friends and soulful music played. Her hips would begin to move back and forth like the ocean, and Bianca found herself getting lost amid it. How could her mother want to shrink something that could make such beautiful waves?

And yet, the women on the magazines her mother bought always had slight hips. There was no expansion there, no waves, no way to hold enough love for the whole world. "I wish my hips would stop before they spread wide as the sea," Bianca said.

After this, Bianca moved to her stomach. Recently, her stomach had become soft. When Bianca sat in some positions, her stomach rolled like dough before her mother made croissants. Bianca remembered liking the softness of her mother's body when she was a child. She felt she could curl up on her mother's middle and stay there forever, enveloped in softness. But the women on her mother's magazines had rigid stomachs. They were flat and ribbed as washing boards and did not look safe to lay on. Bianca began to will the rolls away, "Please give me the energy to do what people do to make their middles soft and hard," she said.

Next, Bianca moved to her chest. She did not even want to think about all the ways a woman's chest could change and how no matter which way it happened, it always seemed to be wrong. She moved quickly to her face, focusing her attention on the roundness of her cheeks. Bianca's mother told her she should smile with fewer teeth so her cheeks wouldn't puff out so far. Bianca had started to smile close-lipped, trying to make her face into a sneer like the mysterious women in the magazines. Sometimes, those women could smile with their teeth because their teeth were bright white, and their cheeks were sucked close to their faces with no puffiness to be seen. But as for Bianca, she could not smile with teeth. This meant she also had to avoid laughing. Bianca began to imagine her cheeks sinking into themselves like holes in the earth, "make my cheeks smaller, and my teeth whiter. Maybe then, I can smile again."

After this, Bianca brought her attention to her nose, imagining it shrinking into just the right angle. It could not be too broad, too large, or curved in a strange way. Then, she imagined her eyes. Compared to the magazines' models, Bianca's eyes looked dull, like a gray sea before a storm. She imagined a tool, swiping across her eyes and making them brighter, like jewels. "Please, make my eyes brighter," she said. Lastly, she imagined her hair. Bianca's mother was always buying new creams, oils, and other products in the attempt to make their hair shine like silk as the women in the magazines did, but it was to no avail. Bianca cringed as she imagined her mother's tears in the bathroom mirror when she tried to curl down the places her hair would not grow silky or lay straight. Bianca began to imagine magic making her hair like shiny silk— "Please, don't let my hair cause my mother to cry. Don't let it make me cry, either."

***

Watching Bianca do her bedtime body scan, her body feeling sad with all the ways she begged it to change, Astrid felt heavy-hearted. She waited outside, waiting for the moment Bianca would fall asleep. "Let the walls of this place melt with magic. Let me transcend them with the intention of blessings." Astrid counted to five while keeping her eyes closed. When she opened them, she was inside Bianca's room, hovering just above the bed. Finally, in sleep, Bianca's face had relaxed.

She no longer squinted her eyes, nor did she frown. Finally, out of the clutch of her mother's eyes on her body, she was free, and she could feel peace. After this, Astrid began to sprinkle gold dust down on Bianca's sleeping body. She would repeat the body scan Bianca had done to herself, but this time, with all new blessed feelings to take into daily life.

Astrid began at Bianca's feet and legs. "These feet are good. They can run, kick a soccer ball, kick in the water to swim, or dance until they are tired on the best nights ever. They are the place where the body roots to the ground, like a tree of great strength. If the feet are the roots, the legs are the trunks. These legs are good. They hold the body strong and support it through the worst of storms. Your legs keep you up and keep you moving, persisting even when things are hard. There is power in these legs that cannot be described in words."

Next, Astrid moved to the hips and sprinkled dust from one bone to the other. "There is an entire world to be explored within these hips. These hips make you an ocean, drawing the world to you with each wave. These hips can dance, they can stretch, and they can hold all the world's magic, right here in your body."

After this, Astrid moved to Bianca's middle-body with the fairy dust. "This body is good. This is the part where the body and the soul are one—that's what makes it feel warm. Everybody is of a different size, and everybody is good. Every soul is the same size, but the size of the temple varies. No matter the size of the body that holds the soul, the beauty is mesmerizing."

Then, Astrid moved up to the chest and arms. "This chest is good. This is where the heart rests. The love in the heart is the entire reason for living. It keeps you alive and loving. The lungs are in this chest too, and the breath in them is the greatest gift you can ever receive. With each breath, life renews itself in fresh moments and changes to experience joy, love more profoundly, and change the world. "These arms are good. These are the arms that hold the ones you love, which paddle you through the sea when you swim, which shoot balls and hold bike handlebars, and greet the ones you love. At the end of the arms are the hands, good hands. They hold the pen from which your poetry flows. They hold on to other people's hands when life becomes hard to live alone. They can help lessen the pain with only a touch.

After this, Astrid moved to the neck and head. "This neck is good. The throat is inside it, and the throat is where you speak from to tell the world your truth. This is where you can speak the truth that the body is only a temple for the soul, and everybody is a good body. This is the place from which you may speak your poetry to the world or sing with music flowing out like honey. When your voice flows out with freedom like a river of honey, it makes the music to the stories of being human. Every voice is important, and every voice is good."

"This head is good. Inside the brain is an oasis of creativity. All the poems you have written and will write in the future are here, waiting to change the world. Your ideas and the things you learn are here. The feelings you experience are here. The brain protects us by telling us what we should do. It creates questions so we can learn more about the world around us. It gives us words to describe the things we feel and ideas for bringing those things alive in the world around us. There is no such thing as a brain with nothing to offer—the brain within everyone's skull has something different and incredible to offer as Knowledge to the world."

After Astrid had finished, she watched a smile spread across Bianca's lips. At last, her body relaxed fully into the mattress, and she slept in a feeling of peace and love for her body and all it had done for her.

There was just one last thing for Astrid to do before she departed. She reached into her knapsack and retrieved dust the color of red rubies. This was the dust of courage, and it was reserved for exceptional occasions. If there was one thing Bianca needed more than anything, it was courage. Astrid began to speak her blessings, raining ruby red dust down onto Bianca's beautiful body.

"May you have the courage to take up space and know you deserve to be there."

"May you have the courage to stand up to your mother, or anyone else who ever sees your body as a container for their opinions or criticisms criticizes. May you tell them, 'my body is everything it needs to be, just as it is. And yours is, too."

"May you have the courage to love your body and yourself with no boundaries. May you care for yourself in the ways only you know how and thank your body for all it does for you. May you thank it

for giving a home to your brain, your heart, and your soul. You are, and always will be, enough."

Millie and the Moon Horse

Part 1: Ordinary Life

"Millie!" Her mother's third call finally cut through the daze of Millie's morning reading. "Get your head out of that book! You haven't eaten a bite of your oatmeal; now you're going to go to school late *and* hungry."

Millie hastily put down her copy of *The Moon Book,* shoveled one final bite of oatmeal into her mouth, and jumped up from the table, dishes in hand. She set them in the sink, glancing once over her shoulder to make sure her mom didn't see her leave them there. Millie stole a look at herself in the reflection on the microwave, stopping for a moment to fix the strands of red hair that had already fallen loose from her braids. Then, she grabbed her yellow-plaid backpack off the hook on the kitchen door, laced up her brown leather combat boots, and opened the front door, calling a final "Bye, mom!" over her shoulder. She started down the block, trying to walk a bit more quickly than usual to take the bus. It was a crisp September morning in the suburban town of Eaglerich, where every house was just a variation of the next. Two things set Millie's home apart from the rest of the places on her block.

The first was the fact that the siding was painted light blue instead of white or gray. The second was that the lawn was not as clean-cut as all the others because Millie's mom refused to use fertilizer on the grass. Millie's favorite place in all of Eaglerich was her backyard, where her mother had planted wildflowers and installed a cast stone fountain with a reflecting pool.

Millie was distracted from thinking about her mother's garden and the cast stone fountain when she saw that her bus had already arrived at the stop. She picked her pace up to a jog, waving a freckled arm so the driver could see her. Breathlessly, Millie climbed onto the bus and began to scan the rows for a place to call her own for these fifteen minutes of peace before arriving at school. Her eyes fell on a seat in the back of the bus, near the window, and she made her way down the aisle, trying to hold her body in close so she wouldn't touch anyone. Once Millie reached her seat, she felt her breath leave her body in a sigh of relief.

She unzipped her yellow-plaid backpack, opened *The Moon Book*, and settled into her seat for fifteen minutes of peace. This morning, however, Millie found herself distracted. Outside the bus window, Millie saw buildings, people, and lawns that all looked the same. Everything about Eaglerich felt too ordinary. Most people lived in the area for a long time, and they felt most comfortable having the same kinds of houses, the same types of jobs, the same types of churches and cars and coffee and everything else. In Eaglerich, success looked like having a home on Eaglerich lake and having your last name well-spoken throughout the town. Millie knew from all of her reading that the world consisted of much more than two-story houses, clean-cut lawns, and Eaglerich Lake, and she hoped one day she would discover it for herself.

***

Millie didn't like school. It wasn't that she didn't enjoy learning; she loved to learn. She didn't like that every book seemed to be a variation of the others at school, and every person seemed to be saying some variation of the same thing about crushes, soccer, or videogames. In Mr. Normandy's class, Millie was seated next to Maxine Walters and Mia Reed. Ever since the start of sixth grade, Maxine and Mia wore the same sparkly *Kiss Me* lip-gloss and passed lists back and forth, ranking every person in the class on a scale of 1-10. The girls updated the list regularly, and while Millie didn't know what factors they used to determine their rankings, she had seen it once. Halfway down the list, next to her name, Millie Maxwell was written: "5/10. She would look better if she wore lip-gloss and didn't have all those freckles!" Maxine and Mia spent most of their time whispering to one another about plans for the weekend. Sometimes, they went to the movies, other times they went to the mall, sometimes they went to the soccer fields to watch other kids from the school play.

Millie wasn't interested in the mall, soccer fields, or lip-gloss, and she was only interested in certain types of movies. But that didn't change the fact that sometimes, Millie wished she had a friend to spend time with on the weekends and pass notes to in class. Millie passed her time at school, making lists of questions in her light pink ring-bound notebook. She wrote questions like: "What does it feel like to eat ice cream on the moon?" "How do other countries see my country?" and "What are the stories I haven't heard?" If Millie had a best friend like Maxine and Mia had each other, she would share the list with them, and they would write all of their questions about the world.

"Quiet, please, everyone! We have a new student in class today that I would like to introduce!" Mr. Normandy shouted. Millie turned her head to see a girl with smooth, dark skin and hair wrapped in a vibrant scarf the sunrise color.

"Will you please tell the class your name?" Mr. Normandy asked.

"My—my name is Claudia. I'm from Angola," The girl murmured.

Millie turned her head to Mr. Normandy's Map of the World that took up half of the wall on the room's right side. She scanned the continent of Africa, trying to find Angola. Millie flipped open her light pink notebook and began to scribble questions. "Where is Angola?" "What language do you speak there?" "What do people in Angola think of my country?" "What is the name of the headscarf, and why do you wear it?" When Claudia came to sit down, Millie smiled at her. "This is my opportunity to learn more about the world," Millie thought to herself, "but I'm too afraid to ask. I'll just keep my questions to myself for now."

Part 2: Arrival of the Moon Horse

When Millie got home from school, her father was gone, and her mother was reading in the den. Millie stole a glance at the book's title "The World of Wildflowers." Behind her ruby-rimmed reading glasses, Millie's mother's eyes were always tired-looking. The lines around her thin mouth drooped down like a wilting leaf. Millie's mother was not the type to ask about her day. If Millie did choose to tell her something about her day, her mother's response was a series of "Oh, I see" and "That's nice, dear." The only thing that brought light to Millie's mother's eyes was gardening. She loved to spend her time outside in the garden, tending to her wildflowers, not having to speak to anyone. Millie wondered if her mother's tiredness and her frustration came from the same place of knowing how much more there was in the world but not knowing how to become a part of it.

Millie went to the kitchen, grabbed herself an apple, then went to the garden to read. Even though it was still warm, Millie couldn't help but remember how soon winter would arrive. All the leaves on the trees would wither up like the lines around her mother's lips, the sky would become gray, and the wildflowers would retreat until the following spring. Millie had to spend as much time outside as she could while it was still warm. She settled into a sun-soaked spot on the grass, opened *The Moon Book*, and did not move until the shadows of evening fell upon the grass.

***

That night after dinner, Millie put on her lavender lace nightgown and sat on her yellow-canopy bed with her moon calendar spread across her lap. Millie had become quite friendly with the Moon, as it was the only place where she felt safe enough to ask her questions and talk about the things that confused her. She felt she owed the Moon for always listening so patiently to her, so she decided to buy a moon calendar to learn more about the Moon's life.

Millie had learned that the Moon has eight phases. The New Moon was the beginning of the phases of the Moon. In this phase, the sun's light shone on the side of the Moon facing the sun. Since it was facing away from earth in this stage, the Moon could not be easily detected in the night sky. Next were the waxing phases: the phases in which the portion of the Earth-side of the Moon is lit by sunlight increases steadily, making the Moon appear slightly bigger and brighter. The three stages of the waxing phases were:

Waxing Crescent (slight edge-lit by the sun), First Quarter (half-lit Moon), and Waxing Gibbous (more of the Moon is illuminated than dark). After these stages, there was the Full Moon, which, according to people worldwide, was the most magical phase of the Moon. In this phase, the Moon's face was utterly bright and formed a full circle, and it rose at almost the same time as the sunset. The final phases were the Waning Phases, which came after the Full Moon. In these phases, the illuminated portion of the Moon's face began to get smaller by night until the New Moon came again. This also came in three phases: The Waning Gibbous (where the illuminated portion is larger than the dark portion but grows smaller every night), Third Quarter (where the Moon is once again half-lit, this time on the left side instead of the right), and Waning Crescent (where the Moon appears as just a sliver in the sky). Out of all the phases, Millie liked the Full Moon best. The world became a magical place when the Moon was full.

As she began to feel her eyelids grow heavier, Millie reached for the lamp on her bedside table. As the yellow glow of the lamp faded from the room, the Moon's milky-white glow replaced it. Millie watched the familiar light dance gently on her walls. Sitting up cross-legged, she lifted a corner of her yellow canopy to see the Moon more clearly.

"Moon, I know I have a pretty good life. But I feel so frustrated sometimes. Why is it so hard for me to find friends to talk to?

Why don't the people around me have more questions about the world? And why am I so afraid to ask the questions I do have?" Millie waited for the answer, but she was met only by the reassuring glow that made her feel listened to. "It frustrates me that people spend so much time talking about ordinary Eaglerich things when there is an entire world out there that we could be asking and learning about. My parents are too tired to talk to me, and I wonder if one day, I might become tired, too."

Millie waited in the solace of the moonlight. She loved the way the Moon held space for her, but sometimes she wished it would only tell her what to do. Why couldn't the Moon give her the strength to ask the questions she wanted to ask out loud? Why couldn't it make her brave enough to talk to Claudia or ask Mr. Normandy about the stories in their sixth-grade history books? "I guess that's all I have for tonight, Moon," Millie said. "I know you get to see the entire world, and you know a lot more about everything than I do. If you think of any advice, I'll be waiting for it."

***

On this particular night, no matter how hard Millie tried to sleep, the questions in her mind kept her awake. Her head buzzed like a beehive, and the feeling that there was something else out there fluttered in her chest like a million butterflies.

Millie felt the only way to calm herself was to become closer to the Moon. Suddenly, she had an idea. Gently, Millie crawled from her bed, tiptoed across the moonlit floorboards, and hoisted herself over the window ledge. She grabbed a branch of the Russian Olive tree growing up against the wall and used it to shimmy down to the yard below. Once her bare toes hit the grass, Millie tiptoed across the yard to her mother's garden. There, in the garden, Millie sat by the cast stone fountain and saw the face of the Moon rippling up close in the pool.

As she listened to the sound of the water and the wind rustling in the wildflower petals, she felt the energy of the Moon reflecting on her face and calming her. Somehow, she felt less alone here, in the garden. Millie basked in the reflection of the Moon until she began to feel her eyelids grow heavy. She stood, stretched her freckled arms towards the sky, and prepared to tiptoe back across the grass towards the Russian Olive tree.

Before Millie could take her first step, she heard the wind begin to change its course, shaking the wildflowers in their place and nearly uprooting them. The water began to splash over the sides of the cast stone fountain, and the light of the Moon on the surface of the water became blinding. Millie was tossed back into the grass with force, and she was entirely blinded by milky moonlight. "What's going on?" Millie called into the light and wind. After several moments, she saw a figure emerging through the light a few yards in front of her. Squinting, Millie saw the flowing mane, broad back, and raring hooves. "Is that... a horse?" she asked.

Millie's question was met by the echo of an angelic, faraway voice. "Millie, I am not just any horse. I am the Moon Horse."

"The Moon Horse?" Millie asked.

"The Moon has heard your calls to her, and on this full Moon, she has sent me to you. I have come to teach you more about the world."

"Are you sure you have the right person?" Millie asked. "I'm just ordinary Millie Maxwell from Eaglerich."

"You speak to the moon every night, do you not?" the Moon Horse asked her.

"Y-yes, I guess I do," Millie said.

"Millie Maxwell, it is you the Moon has sent me to. It is an accomplishment to understand that there is far more in this world than what you see in your city, your neighborhood, and your own family. For the next three nights of the Full Moon, you must meet me right here in the garden. I will come to you, and we will go to other corners of the world the Moon shines its face upon. There, you will see the lives of other children like yourself, and you will understand how much more there is to life."

Millie did not know what to say, so she simply nodded in agreement. With that, she felt the force of the winds kick up, and a milky light blinded her. Within moments, the Moon Horse had vanished. Millie rubbed her eyes and began to run her fingertips along her face and arms to ensure that she was genuinely standing there. What if this had all just been a dream? Dazed, Millie started across the grass towards the house again. She clambered up the Russian Olive tree and through the open window. She tiptoed across the floorboards to her yellow-canopy bed, where she laid down, staring up at the ceiling and trying to process all she had just seen. No matter what, Millie would do what the Moon Horse said. Tomorrow night, she would go to the garden, and she would wait.

Part 3: The First Visit

The following day at school, Millie could think of nothing but the moon horse. She continued to ask herself if what she had seen the night before had been a dream. How could it be real? Millie was not concerned with Mia and Maxine's conversations, nor Mr. Normandy's lectures. She noticed Claudia's headscarf, this time in shades of teals and purple, with yellow accents. But even that was not enough to keep her attention for long. Millie rushed home from school at the end of the day and spent her afternoon willing the sun to go down. She could hardly even focus on *The Moon Book*.

That night after dinner, Millie took a shower and put on her lavender lace nightgown. She began to pace the room, looking at the clock every few moments to see how close it was to 10:00. That was when the Moon Horse had met her last night, and she needed to be sure she wasn't late. Suddenly, Millie had an idea. If she was going to see the world, she'd better have some questions available. Maybe she would even find the answers to some of the questions already written in her book. She snuck down the hall towards the kitchen where her backpack hung on the door hook, took out her light pink notebook, and dashed back upstairs as quickly as possible.

Finally, after what felt like an eternity, the clock struck 9:45. Millie decided now was the time to get out of bed and go to the garden so she could be sure not to be late. Before heading out the window and down the Russian Olive tree, she grabbed her light pink notebook and a pen, tucking them in the lavender lace nightgown near her hip. She hurried down the side of the house and tiptoed across the garden to the meeting place. She waited there among the wildflowers and the cast stone fountain, listening for the wind to change direction and pick up its force. Sure enough, after a few minutes, Millie heard the same rushing sound through the wildflowers and saw the water in the cast stone fountain begin to leap into the air. The milky white light blinded her, and this time, she did not feel afraid.

"Millie," the familiar, angelic voice echoed, "I'm so happy to see you."

"Moon Horse," Millie spoke timidly, "Where are we going? And how are we going to get there?"

Millie watched an ethereal smile spread across the moon horse's radiant face. "I can't tell you where we are going. But here, climb on my back and hold tight to my mane."

The moon horse leaned forward on her front legs so Millie could climb on. Her back was smooth and muscled, and her mane felt like silk between Millie's fingertips.

"Ready?" she asked, turning her shining lavender eyes over her shoulder to glance at Millie. "Ready," Millie responded, tightening her grip on the silken mane.

All of a sudden, Millie felt the moon horse leave the ground.

There was an incredible rush of air all around them, blowing Millie's hair back and causing her heart to race. All she could see around her was a mirage of flying colors, mostly shades of blue, white, and purple. She could not make out where she was; all she could do was grip the Moon Horse tighter. Millie lost track of time in the vacuum of their journey, and she was jolted back to reality only once the Moon Horse's hooves hit solid ground.

***

The first thing Millie noticed was the heavy heat of the sun on her shoulders. Wherever she was, it was no longer night. The dust cleared to make way for a view of a bustling street crowded with cars, motorcycles, painted buses, and what appeared as carts on bicycle wheels. The buildings were stacked like leaning towers with small windows clad in drying laundry of all colors. Millie heard cars honking and vendors selling fruits, scarves, street food, and other goods all around her. Many women wore jangling bracelets, dangling earrings, and studs of diamonds or gold rings in their noses. Many people's feet were bare or clad only by sandals, and they were caked in the hot brown dust. Millie saw goats on ropes and cows wandering free in the crowded streets.

Whenever a cow crossed the road or stopped to graze, everyone else stopped to give it space. Never in her life had Millie been on the street full of so much life as this one.

"Moon Horse," Millie spoke, "where are we?"

"We are on the street of Colaba in Mumbai," the moon horse replied.

"Where is Mumbai?" Millie asked.

"In India," said the moon horse, "this is our first stop."

Millie saw a beautiful girl with thick, ebony hair down to her waist as they trotted down the road. The girl's hair was braided and tied at the end with a magenta ribbon, detailed in gold to match the earrings that dangled nearly to her neck like golden chandeliers. Millie raised her hand to wave to the girl, but the girl did not react.

"She can't see you, Millie," the moon horse said, "we are invisible here."

The farther they trotted, the more Millie began to feel the afternoon heat weighing down upon her. "How much farther?" she asked tentatively.

"Just a little while longer," the moon horse responded.

They began to trot up a staircase on the side of a hillock to a tower of limestone and marble, glinting brilliantly in the hot afternoon sun.

They trotted beneath an archway at the front and watched people going in and out. Many of the people walking in and out of the temple had small red dots on their foreheads, just between their eyebrows. "That red dot is called a *bindi*," said the moon horse, "it sits on the third-eye chakra, which is believed to be the body's center of inner wisdom.

Followers of the Hindu tradition believe that people have three eyes. The first two are the ones we see on people's faces every day—those that see the outside world. The third one is located right between them, and its purpose is to focus inward towards the true essence, or God." Millie was fascinated. In Eaglerich, most people put God in a box. They did not care how the rest of the world saw God, and they probably did not know much about reaching God through a third-eye.

"The bindi can also be worn by Indian women to symbolize marriage in the Hindu and Jain traditions. It is believed to bring the woman prosperity in marriage and her family unit," the moon horse explained. Millie had never heard anything like this, and she wanted to know more. "Moon Horse, can you tell me about this tower?" she asked.

"This is the *Balbunath Temple,* one of the oldest temples in all of Mumbai. In the Hindu tradition, there are hundreds of Gods, and they all represent different living things. The Balbunath Temple was created for the Hindu god *Shiva* in the form of the Lord of the Babul Tree. In Hinduism, three gods are believed to be a part of the creation, maintenance, and destruction of the world. Shiva is a very passionate god and is seen as a source of both good and evil, capable of both destroying and reconstructing the world," the Moon Horse explained.

"Who are the other two gods?" Millie asked.

"The first of them is *Brahma*, who is believed to be the creator of the universe. He has four arms and four heads. The second is *Vishnu,* the God of restoration and bringing balance back to the world. He is a bearer of light, often associated with the sun."

"Wow," Millie said, "I like thinking there could be so many gods, all responsible for different things." She glanced at the intricate stone of the building and the beautiful people wandering in and out.

As if reading Millie's mind, the Moon Horse said, "You may enter the sanctum. But if you wish to do so, there are some specific things you must know."

"I'm ready to hear them," Millie said.

"A sanctum is a place for serenity, peace, and emptying your mind. It is a place where you allow yourself to come entirely into the present moment in your body and be guided back to your true self. You must move with respect, allowing the space to move you, teach you, bring you peace, and feel the true Godliness inside yourself."

"I think I can do that," Millie said.

"You can," the Moon Horse said, "just sit comfortably, close your eyes, and let the atmosphere of the temple surround you as if you have emerged in the sea. Let yourself emerge in the sea of mindfulness and possibility."

***

Millie saw a girl around her age inside the temple, draped in cream and gold, with gold bangles on her wrists and hoops dangling from her ears.

She entered the temple with fluid movements, like a river of milk and honey. Millie watched the girl walk to space on the floor just next to her. She looked at Millie with gentle, knowing eyes.

Her dark lashes fluttered shut, like closing gates as she entered another world. Millie watched the girl's face give way to pure softness, a smile on her lips that said she could dream of being nowhere else. At that moment, this girl looked purely content, resting in what was and wishing for nothing else. She sat with crossed legs, one bare foot settled on top of the other. Her palms were turned upwards towards the sky; thumb gently balanced on her index finger. Millie shifted, crossing her legs and positioning her fingers the same way. Slowly, Millie let her auburn eyelashes close, breathing in as she began her journey.

As Millie sat, she frequently found herself drawn away from the moment by thoughts. Could it be that this was all a dream? Why had she never heard anything like this before? How could this girl her age seem so natural as she entered into the present moment with peace and joy? What was this Godliness inside oneself that the Moon Horse referred to? Each time a thought arose, Millie let it be and continued to breathe. After a while, she began to feel something light and warm rising within her.

The warmth began at the base of her belly and spread up her spine, across her chest, wrapping around her heart like a hug. She felt it pulsing through her throat and up through her face, relaxed now, into her head. It was as if a string was attached to her head, pulling her upwards towards a place of holiness, of magic, of pure satisfaction. Millie sat with this feeling of light within her, allowing her body to float, as if she, too, were on a river of milk and honey. When Millie's eyes fluttered back awake to the world, she still felt the light in her. Everything around her was the most beautiful thing she had ever seen, and she wished to be nowhere else. "This," Millie thought to herself, "this is a feeling I wish to carry with me for the rest of my life."

Suddenly, Millie saw only darkness, intermingled with swirling colors of light. She felt a thump, and when her eyelashes fluttered open again, she was back in her bed; pale moonlight shining through her white canopy like an omen. Millie stared at the light for a while until she felt her eyelids grow heavy and fell into a deep sleep.

***

The following morning, Millie woke as she always did to her mother's sound in the kitchen. She wondered if last night had truly happened—had she been to a temple in Mumbai? Millie rose from the bed, but she had an idea before going to the bathroom to shower. Millie grabbed a pillow from her bed and placed it on the floor. She sat down, crossing one leg over the other, and gently balancing her hands on her knees, palms up, index finger meeting thumb. She let her eyelids close and began to breathe, allowing the beauty, joy, and satisfaction of this new day to fill her lungs. Millie let them smile softly as thoughts arose as each thought appeared and melted away with her breaths.

When Millie opened her eyes, the warm light was radiating through her body again. She proceeded to shower and dress; then she went down to the kitchen where her mother was standing at the sink, sipping her coffee with exhaustion as she stared out the window at nothing in particular. "Mom," Millie spoke timidly, "I love you." Millie saw her mother's tired eyes spring open a bit farther in surprise. Then, a soft smile spread across her lips, making her look a little younger and almost happy. "I love you too, Millie," she said.

On the way to school that morning, everything seemed more beautiful. The sun rippled through the leaves, making them like green emeralds or the entrance to another world. Every person Millie saw looked more beautiful too, as she thought of how each of them had a story. Everyone was beautiful—the mailman with his blue button-up shirt who whistled to himself, the woman in the faded pink nightgown watering her lilies, the motorcyclist with art on his arms, the bus driver with her silver braid who said "Good morning," to every student. The city passed by the window in whirls of curiosity and human life and the possibility of a new day with a million different stories unfolding within it. Millie felt the light inside her pulsing with the magic of it all. She closed her eyes, breathed in, and said, "Thank you." She didn't know to whom she was expressing gratitude, but she knew it was going to the place that connected her to everyone else in her city and across the globe, and for her, that was enough.

Part 4: The Second Visit

When Millie got home from school that day, she returned to the garden to ponder everything she had experienced once again. She was perplexed by the events of the night before, still unsure whether or not she had dreamt of them. Regardless, the fullness in her heart lasted throughout the day, and she found herself noticing more beautiful things than she usually did. She saw the jungle of colors on Claudia's headscarf and felt her soul jump with joy each time her eyes settled on a new one. She had made eye contact with Claudia, too, and the two girls had smiled at each other. On the way home, Millie noticed the way the trees danced on the wind, the way the cream-colored butterflies fluttered by, the squirrels scampered around with their acorns, and the neighbors drank lemonade on their porches, trimmed their hedges, rode their bicycles, or grilled out on their decks. As they sat in the garden that afternoon, Millie felt excitement at how many opportunities existed for her in this world. She relaxed in the afternoon sun and prayed the Moon Horse would come to her again that night.

Later that night, after she had eaten dinner and gotten ready for bed, Millie could hardly contain herself as she laid awake in bed. She brimmed with anticipation for the Moon Horse to come to her for the second night of the Full Moon. As she tossed and turned in bed, Millie grew impatient. Finally, the clock struck 9:45.

Once again, Millie crawled from her bed and grabbed her light pink notebook and pen from the bedside table. She scurried down the trunk of the

Russian Olive Tree until her bare feet hit the dew-wet grass. She tiptoed across the garden, which was glowing white in the milky light of the Full Moon. Once she reached the meeting place, she sat near the cast stone fountain meeting places and waited. She watched the wildflowers, waiting to see their dance change with the forceful change of the wind's direction.

Just as she began to wonder if it would not happen, after all, she saw the water of the cast stone fountain splash into the air in a majestic stream, and the wildflowers changed into a dance of larger movements, accompanied by the rushing sound through their petals. Millie's eyes became blinded by the white light, and she felt her heart leap for joy just as the water in the fountain did.

"Good evening, Young Millie," the Moon Horse greeted her.

"Good evening, Moon Horse," Millie responded.

"Tell me, how was your day today?" the Moon Horse asked.

"Oh, it was lovely. It was like I saw my whole life in a brand new light. I felt this fullness in my heart all day, and everything around me looked all the more beautiful," Millie answered.

The Moon Horse did not say anything, only nodded back with the same ethereal smile. Then, the Moon Horse spoke again, "Well, I think you'll be changed by the place we are traveling today as well. Here, climb on my back, and don't forget to grasp tightly to my mane." The Moon Horse leaned down, and

Millie climbed on, with much greater ease this time than she had the night before. Millie felt a sense of peace fill her as she felt the smoothness of the Moon Horse's muscled back and the silky softness of her mane.

"Ready?" the Moon Horse asked, turning her shining lavender eyes over her shoulder again to ensure Millie was situated. "Ready," Millie responded, and she felt her stomach begin to feel as if it were inhabited by thousands of cream-colored butterflies, ready for what would come next.

All at once, Millie felt her body begin to rise from the garden ground. She felt the familiar rush of cold air, which blew her hair back and made the butterflies in her stomach flutter faster, all the way up to her heart. The mirage of flying colors reappeared, and she noticed shades of blue, white, and purple she had never seen before. She kept her grip on the moon horse as they flew through the universe at top speed, gliding towards wherever the next destination would be.

Once again, in the vacuum of the journey, Millie could not keep track of time. She was far too mesmerized by the colors and shapes of the universe whizzing by and the air blowing back her hair with great force to think of anything else.

Suddenly, she felt the jolt of the Moon Horse's hooves, hitting the solid ground again.

"We're here," the Moon Horse spoke.

***

Millie looked around. On one side of her, there were only trees for as far as she could tree. Millie was sure she had never seen so many trees in her life; they hung thick and dense over a jungle which she imagined contained more creatures than she could ever name. To Millie's other side, there was a river the color of copper. It stretched across so wide she could hardly see the other end, and it looked more like a lake than a river. Along the banks of the river was an odd mud the color of red brick. The air was thick, warm, and wet, and it felt heavy on Millie's freckled cheeks. The scent of fish, trees, and red earth flooded Millie's nostrils. Where could she be?

"This is the Amazon Rainforest," the moon horse told her, "Have you heard of it?"

Millie had heard of the rainforest. In class, they learned about the rainforest creatures, that the Amazon River was the longest river on the planet, and that the Amazon rainforest was called the "lungs of the world" because of all the trees. She knew there were animals like pythons, sloths, poisonous dart frogs, and giant spiders. On the zoo's class field trip, the class had the chance to visit an exhibit that was supposed to look like a rainforest, but this was indeed much different from that. "Yes," Millie answered the moon horse, "I have heard of the Amazon rainforest. What I know most is about the river, all the trees, and the creatures that exist almost nowhere else on earth."

"That's right," the Moon Horse said with a nod, "But this place is much more than a natural wonderland. People are living here, too. And the people who live in the rainforest live much differently than people who live in cities like the one you're from. These people are the natives. They were here, and in your country, long before anyone else got there.

They know the secrets of the earth that nobody else knows, and they live in harmony with the plants, the trees, the river, the sky, and everything in sight." No sooner had the Moon Horse said this, Millie saw a group of children running out of the thick forest towards the riverbank.

The children were wearing brown clothes fastened around their waists, and they were yelling and laughing in a language Millie didn't understand. Behind the children came several women, all of them wearing only brown skirts around their waists and thick braids in their hair. All of the women in children had their faces painted with black designs and the earth's mud-red color near the river.

Millie watched as the children ran into the river and began to swim around, floating on their backs, kicking their legs, and splashing one another. The women entered too, and sat in the cold water, washing as they chatted. Millie did not speak; she simply watched these people in front of her, splashing in the river and being at one with the planet that was their home.

***

After the women and children finished their bath in the river, they began to head up the bank again and into the undergrowth. "Come on," the Moon Horse spoke, "we will follow them." As the Moon Horse trotted through the undergrowth, Millie kept her head down to avoid getting hit by any of the swinging branches, or worse, a creature that could be lurking. As they trotted, the Moon Horse began to educate Millie.

"About 1 million Native people are living in the Amazon region. They are divided into 400 tribes spread across their territories. Each tribe has a culture and language that are unique to that particular tribe," the Moon Horse said. Millie was fascinated. She could not believe that the Native people had spread out in so many different directions and that they each had elements of language and culture that no other Native people shared.

"As you can see with these villagers, most Native people inhabit villages by the rivers. In these communities, the river is a source of life. It is what makes the ground fertile and makes it possible for vegetables and fruits to grow. Some of the most popular crops in this region are manioc, corn, bananas, and beans," said the Moon Horse, "The people here know how to take great care of the land, make it fertile, and gather crops to feed the village."

Millie thought of her mother's tomatoes in the summer and how much attention it took to tend to them. Her mother had to watch to make sure they received enough sunlight and water and prayed that the weather would not be too dry, cold, or stormy. If the weather was bad, the crop was ruined. Millie could not even imagine the skill it would take, and how nerve-wracking it might be, to have an entire lifestyle and the feeding of a village dependent on crops.

"As you can see, we are essentially out in the middle of nowhere. You have to take a boat to get here from the nearest city, and even that is several hours away. There are no grocery stores or restaurants here," the Moon Horse explained. "These societies are hunter-gatherer societies, which means a major way they get food is through hunting, fishing, and foraging for foods like nuts and berries that grow naturally here. There is endless wildlife available here, but it takes a lot of skill to catch it. When the tribesmen go out to fish, they create poison out of local plants. This poison shocks the fish, making it impossible for them to swim away. It is poisonous to the fish, but people can eat it with no problem."

"And hunting?" Millie asked, "what methods do they use to do that?" "That depends on where you go," the Moon Horse answered. "Some tribes use the traditional bow and arrows or hunting spears. Some tribes use blowguns with poisonous darts. And there a few tribes who use the more modern technology of shotguns." The Moon Horse explained that it could take weeks for the huntsmen to bring the game back to the village, and because of that, it was always a treat when it happened. "The staple food of the village is manioc, a root vegetable which is grown on the fertile ground down by the river," the Moon Horse explained, "Manioc is toxic when it is first harvested, and the women spend many hours removing the toxins from the mixture to make it safe to eat."

Millie noticed they had been walking for quite some time, and there was still no village in sight. "Is it normal for us to have to walk this far from the river?" she asked nervously. "Perfectly normal," answered the moon horse, "the tribes live deep in the forest far away from the rivers. They have to make long treks to fish, harvest crops, and wash."

"Do they stay in the same place forever?" Millie asked, thinking of how common it was for people to move around a lot back where she came from. "Some tribes are nomadic, which means they move. When a tribe moves, it is usually to find better food sources or escape natural conditions that make it hard to stay. Tribes used to move around much more than they do now in search of food. However, in recent years, most tribes remain in their villages and do not move anywhere new.

This is becoming a problem, though, as more people from the outside are discovering the tribes and trying to bring their people into the cities. Another problem is that the Amazon rainforest is in danger. Sometimes there are extensive fires that break out, forcing tribes out of their homes. The river is becoming polluted too, with the trash thrown overboard on boats and the pollution from factories worldwide. This water is another dangerous thing to the Amazonian tribes." Millie stayed quiet for a moment, shuddering at how scary it would be to have to flee everything she had ever known because the forest was burning, or to bathe in the same river and rely on it for food all her life, only to have it turn into something dangerous.

Finally, they arrived at the village. Millie looked around and saw children running all around. Women bustled back and forth, carrying baskets. Many of the buildings had no walls, only a thatched roof supported by wooden beams. Beneath several of the thatched roofs, women worked, pounding manioc into flour to eat. Scattered throughout the village, several buildings were longer and looked a bit like logs. "These are communal buildings where people live together. Everything is focused on the community here," the Moon Horse said, "they share everything too. No one hoards their resources. The beauty, knowledge, food, and medicine that belongs to one tribe member belongs to the others as well."

***

Suddenly, Millie was startled to hear the pounding of a drum. She turned around and saw people running to gather beneath a thatched-roof communal space.

She and the Moon Horse drew nearer to the outside of the space and watched as the tribe members began to join hands for a group dance. They started to dance in a circle, to chant, and sing. "Song and dance are used to build a sense of community and as an offering of prayer," the Moon Horse said, "Every tribe has songs, dances, and crafts which are unique to that particular tribe."

As she watched the people dance, she felt their footsteps in rhythm with the beat of her own heart, and their chanting made her feel as if her body could become transcendent. "Moon Horse," she spoke, "I feel something deeply spiritual happening within me." The moon horse smiled. "To the Amazonian tribes, this rainforest is a deeply sacred place. Every flower, plant, and animal in this place is believed to contain its spirit. The Native people believe that humans should live in harmony with nature, moving with it, never wasting resources, and not doing anything to disturb the natural order of things. They have a deep reverence for every plant and creature in this place. They know more about the earth than almost anyone else, including how to use plants that exist in nature as medicine to heal many medical conditions."

Millie was shocked and found herself eager to know more about this healing. She could not believe there were so many plants in the world that could heal wounds and make people feel better when sick. "The belief that all living things have a spirit within them is called animism, and it is a practice followed in the culture of most Native Amazonians," said the Moon Horse, "When members of the tribe fall ill, are injured, or are dealing with another challenge, there are people who can use the power of the spirits to heal them.

These people are called Shamans, and they are healers appointed by the tribe. Sometimes, they will disappear into the forest for days, or even weeks, to bring themselves in touch with the spirits necessary to heal and protect their tribe from enemies." "Do the Shamans know the same things doctors know?" Millie asked.

"Oh, yes," said the Moon Horse, "As much, and in some cases, even more. There have been researchers who study these tribes and determine that the Shamans understand some of even the most complicated medical conditions."

Millie and the Moon Horse remained in the village until the sun began to set, casting shades of pink, lavender, and orange on the copper water beyond the forest. Millie watched in awe as the villagers gathered in a circle and began to share a meal.

"Millie," the Moon Horse spoke, her voice solemn, "it is essential that you know that Native people are not safe in many places in the world. The rest of the world, especially people who live in the cities and want to clear places like this to find more oil and other resources to be rich, often come into these communities and force people out of their homes. Sometimes they have to go into the cities, where they are forced into very poor conditions and have a lot of trouble finding jobs that pay, adequate shelter, and enough to eat. The oil industry is a considerable threat to these communities.

People clear large areas of these forests to find the oil reserves underneath. This often pollutes the land and poisons the waterways, making it difficult to survive. The trees that are not cut down sometimes burn away when fires break out. The hotter the earth gets, the more fires break out, and the more villages are destroyed. It is up to your generation to speak up for Native people, to protect their resources, and let them live undisturbed by the outside world. Not only that, but the world could learn something from them, too. There is so much to learn from the Native people about how to live at one with nature and find the beauty, spirituality, and healing power within it."

The two trotted back to the bank of the river, where the reflection of the setting sun was fading to shades of purple and blue, and stars appeared like diamonds above the thick shadows of the trees. "Let's do something before we go," the Moon Horse said, "Close your eyes. Breathe in the scent of this place—the glory of nature. Allow the spirits of the animals, plants, and people you have seen to fill you. When you exhale, open your heart in prayer for the healing of the people from this community. Ask the spirits to watch over you and lead you in the ways you, too, can protect the earth. There is only one planet, and we all have lessons to learn about how to care for it."

Millie was flooded with darkness after she exhaled, intermingled with the same swirling rays of light in all colors. After a while, she felt her body thump down, and her eyelashes fluttered open to reveal she was back in her bed. The pale moonlight shone through her white canopy, and it was as if she could hear the voice of the moon singing peacefully, coaxing her into a deep sleep.

***

Part 5: The Final Visit

The following morning when Millie awoke, she felt a deep sense of gratitude for the warmth of the sun filtering through her white canopy and warming her pillow. She got up, ate breakfast, and told her mother she loved her again on the way out the door. As she walked to school, her heartfelt light as she took even greater notice of the trees stretching over her street, the blueness of the sky with clouds of every shape, and the flowers growing in front of people's houses. She saw animals too—cats on windowsills, birds swooping through the air at various heights, the same cream-colored butterflies and squirrels with acorns in their mouths, and people walking their dogs. Millie smiled to herself as she imagined the spirits within each of these living things. Suddenly, Millie felt a sense of safety and transcendence, as if she was a part of a divine dance with the world around her.

That afternoon at school, when Claudia and Millie made eye contact, Millie waved hello. Claudia waved back, flashing Millie a shy smile, before turning back around in her seat. Throughout the day, Millie continued to find her eyes drawn outside the window to the playground and the neighborhood beyond, imagining the thousands of spirits that might exist within her city.

When she arrived back home that day after school, Millie went straight to the garden. She stretched her body out in the grass, lush and warm from the sun. She felt the sun on her skin, smelt the sweetness of the wildflowers in her nose, felt the tickle of the breeze, and heard the chirping of the birds. She breathed it all in, inhaling healing thoughts for nature and exhaling blessings and prayers for healthier earth that would always be this beautiful and sacred.

Before dinner, she took her pen and pink journal and wrote these prayers and blessings for the earth in her notebook. Then, she added prayers for protection over the Native Amazonian people and offered a prayer of gratitude for all they did to protect the earth.

***

That night after dinner, Millie practically skipped up the stairs. She showered and put on her lavender lace nightgown, then spent about an hour pacing back and forth on her bedroom floor as she waited for the clock to strike 9:45. She had seen the Moon Horse enough times now that she imagined it had to be real, and she couldn't wait to see where tonight's adventures would take them. Would they visit another area of the world? How did the children live in the areas of the globe Millie had yet to experience?

Finally, the clock struck 9:45. Millie once again grabbed her notebook and pen and scampered across the bedroom floor to her window. She wedged her body through and scurried down the trunk of the Russian Olive Tree, then dashed across the yard until she reached the cast stone fountain.

She sat near the edge of the fountain, imagining the spirits that could be within each type of wildflowers in the garden. She became so busy, she was caught off guard when the direction of the wind changed, the flowers began to jolt every which way, and she felt a cold splash of water from the fountain land on her arm. Once again, her eyes were overtaken by blinding white light, and her heart began to pound and dance in every direction, just as the flowers did.

An angelic voice thundered over the garden. "Hello, Millie.

Are you ready for our third and final night of Full Moon adventures?"

"Yes, I am," Millie answered, "Where are we going tonight?"

"I can't tell you," responded the Moon Horse, "But I do think you'll be surprised for what's in store. Come on, now, hop on."

The Moon Horse bent down and, as if by second nature, Millie swung her body onto the smooth, muscled back and gripped the silk of the Moon Horse's main between her anxious fingers. She felt the familiar rising of her body and the cold air blowing her hair and making every nerve in her body feel alive. The mirage of colors appeared again, this time even more vibrant than the nights before. She held on tight and was shocked when the journey ended much sooner than she expected. They landed with a thump. Millie rubbed her eyes and looked around, confused at the fact that it still appeared to be nighttime in whichever place they had come to.

"Moon Horse," she inquired, "aren't we going to another area of the world?"

"This is another area of the world," the Moon Horse answered. As the two began to walk down the street, Millie felt even more perplexed. There were no temples, rivers, jungles, or cows. Only trees looked like those in her neighborhood and apartment buildings that looked like those in her city. The street was quiet because it was late, and she did not see anyone out on their porches.

Suddenly, they arrived at a squarish apartment with brown bricks and chipping paint around the windowsills. "Here we are," said the Moon Horse. Millie furrowed her brow in confusion as the Moon Horse began to walk gracefully up the concrete staircase. "Moon Horse, what are you doing? We can't go into someone else's home, can we?"

"Millie," the Moon Horse answered, "we do not disturb anyone on these journeys. You see, although we can see them, they cannot see us. We will go inside this apartment to see what is happening there, but the people inside will not notice us, and we will not invade their privacy."

The two continued through the double doors of the apartment and began up seven flights of stairs. When they reached the top, the Moon Horse continued to walk down the hallway until they reached the fourth door on the left. She stopped and told Millie to hold tight to her mane and close her eyes.

When Millie opened her eyes, they were inside the living room of a dimly lit apartment with bare walls and a sagging, dark green couch. Millie could see the reflections of other apartment windows on the block from the large living room window, and beyond that, the silhouette of a city skyline. She could not tell which city it was. On the apartment floor was a small boy in red striped pajamas, watching a cartoon about dinosaurs on the TV. Suddenly, a young girl's voice echoed from the kitchen. "Jimmy, go wash up and then come eat supper!"

The Moon Horse led Millie into the kitchen, where a girl not much older than her stood, stirring a single can of chicken noodle soup in a pot and bouncing a baby on her hip. The girl moved to the cupboard and retrieved baby formula and a bottle. She stirred the mixture into the bottle with some water, then began heating the bottle in the microwave, repeatedly checking the temperature on her wrist. When the baby started to cry, she bounced her and started a chorus of "shhh, shhh, shhh." The little boy in the red striped pajamas came into the kitchen and sat down. The young girl served him a small bowl of soup, along with several stale saltine crackers. She sat down at a chair across from him, feeding the baby her bottle.

"Jimmy," the girl spoke, "have you finished your homework for today?" The little boy stared down into his chicken noodle soup, refusing to make eye contact with her. "I don't have any today," he said meekly. The girl raised her eyebrows. "Jimmy, I know that isn't true. You've been practicing counting and making your letters all week, and I know today is no exception. After dinner, I'll put Josie down, and then I want you to bring it to me, okay?" The little boy nodded and continued to spoon soup into his mouth.

"That's Janie," the Moon Horse explained, "she's your age. Every day she wakes up at 5:30 to make breakfast for Jimmy and Josie, her younger siblings. Jimmy is six, and Josie is one-and-a-half. After Janie wakes up, she makes Josie's bottle and starts breakfast for herself and Jimmy. Then she goes to wake Jimmy up and helps him get ready for school. They all have breakfast together and leave the house by 6:30, so they have time to get Josie to her daycare down the street before Jimmy and Janie catch the 7:00 bus to school."

Millie cringed at the idea of waking up at 5:30, and she couldn't imagine having to wake up two younger siblings and get them to school all by herself. "Don't they have a mommy or a daddy to help?" Millie asked. "Their mommy works night shifts at the supermarket down the street. She doesn't get home until almost 5:00 in the morning every day, so she is too tired to help. And on some days, she doesn't get to come home until even later," the Moon Horse answered. "What about their daddy?" asked Millie. "They all have different dads, and none of them come around much," said the Moon Horse, "it's mostly just the three of them, left to figure things out."

"How does Janie focus on school? And does she have time to get her homework done?" Millie asked with concern." Janie is very studious. She works hard in school and tries her best to get all her homework done. She stays up late every night after putting Jimmy and Josie to bed, and she tries to finish all her assignments.

When she can't figure out how to do something, she can't ask her mother, so she takes it into school and tries to talk with her teachers early to figure out what's missing. Janie has goals of going to college and making enough money as a nurse to support her mom and siblings. Sometimes, though, she is so tired that she misses assignments or begins to fall asleep in class."

***

Millie watched as Janie cleared the table and took the baby to the bathroom. She bathed her little sister and told Jimmy to start on his homework, but he resumed watching cartoons on the living room floor. Janie washed her sister tenderly, singing songs as she did. Once she finished, Millie watched her dress, her sister in a fresh diaper and pajamas. She went down the hall to a bedroom where all three children slept. There was a sagging futon which Jimmy and Janie shared, and a worn crib in the corner for Josie.

Janie walked around the room, walking, swaying, and singing, until eventually, her sister's crying stopped, and she drifted off to sleep. Janie lifted her sister into the crib, then tiptoed out of the room back to the living room.

Once she arrived and saw Jimmy watching cartoons, she crossed her arms sternly. "Jimmy, it's getting late. Go get your homework right now, or we won't have time for a story before bed." The little boy leaped up and ran to the kitchen to retrieve his school bag. The two sat on the green couch for the next thirty minutes while Janie patiently helped her brother add numbers and make the letters that spelled out the words "bug," "bag," and "big." Once they were finished, Janie told her brother to take a shower. "Make sure you wash behind your ears!" she yelled as he went down the hall.

Once Jimmy had disappeared into the bathroom, Millie watched Janie sit for a moment with her head in her hands. Her eyes sagged, and she massaged her temples as if trying to wake herself up for the night of homework that still laid ahead. Eventually, she raised her head again and began to do her history homework while waiting for Jimmy. After Jimmy got out of the shower, he came back out and curled up on the green couch next to his sister. In his hand, he held a worn copy of the children's book, "Goodnight, Moon." This was one of Millie's favorites.

She listened to Janie read the book in a voice so soothing it almost made Jimmy fall asleep on her shoulder. After she was finished, the little boy was so close to sleep that Janie picked him up and carried him to the futon in their bedroom. She tucked him in and went back to the living room to finish her homework. Millie watched Janie working on her history homework—brow furrowed in concentration. She then went on to her arithmetic, which she could not figure out how to finish. It was late, but Janie didn't think she could sleep. Her brain was too busy. She took out a piece of notebook paper and began to scribble a list under the headline "My Questions."

1. Will I make it to college one day?
2. Will I ever meet my father?
3. Will it ever become more comfortable to sleep?
4. Will I be able to help my mom one day?
5. Does Jimmy know we don't have any money?

6. Will Jimmy be happy when he grows up?
7. Will Jimmy do well in school?
8. What will I do if Jimmy struggles?
9. Will Josie live a more comfortable life than Jimmy, and I have?
10. Will Josie be happy?

The stress was rising so high, Janie had to figure out something to do to calm down. She stood up from the couch and walked across the room to a basket underneath the TV.

She retrieved a smudged book of watercolor paper and a palette of watercolor paints, which one of the art teachers had given her. Millie watched as Janie's hand began to glide in graceful movements, creating a scene of a mountain meadow on the paper in front of her. As she painted, her face relaxed, and Millie could feel the worry melting away. "Janie is an artist," the Moon Horse explained to Millie, "she does it when she needs to relax." Millie was at a loss for words for the beauty of the painting Janie made. "Does she get recognition at school? Does she have lessons?" Millie asked.

"Several teachers have recognized her talent, but when they suggest lessons or art club to her, she says she can't because she has to study. The adults at school don't know that Janie comes home every day, meets Jimmy at the bus stop, picks up Josie from daycare, comes home to tidy up the house, make dinner, bathe the children, help Jimmy with his homework, and put both him and Josie to bed. The adults at school don't know that Janie hardly ever sees her mother or that she worries day in and day out about what would happen if Jimmy got on the wrong bus, if Josie got sick at daycare, or if she,

Janie, did not pass one of her classes. She simply tells them she is too busy to put extra time into painting." Millie felt her heart sink in hearing this, and she began to wonder about her classmates. How much of their lives did she not know?

After a while of painting, the girl carefully replaced her supplies and laid the mountain meadow painting on the table to dry. She shuffled across the floor to the bathroom to get ready for bed herself. Once she was ready, she went to double-check the door was locked and that the kitchen was clean. Then she returned to the bedroom and laid down, exhausted, on the futon next to her brother. As Janie tossed and turned, her eyes came to rest on the Moon, shining through the window. Millie was surprised to see Janie begin speaking to the Moon in the same way that she did every night. Janie let out all of her worries, praying that the Moon would guide her, protect her, and help her be the person she should be.

At that moment, Millie realized she had much more in common with other people than she had ever known. No matter what people's lives looked like or what challenges they faced at home, everybody needed a way to calm down with things they enjoyed. Everyone had worries, just like she did, and everyone looked to a force larger than themselves to give them guidance and protection and help them live the lives they were meant to live. Suddenly, the world felt so much smaller, and despite their differences, Millie thought that she shared a heart with Janie.

***

Millie turned to face the Moon Horse again. "Where are we going now?" she asked. "This is it, Millie," the Moon Horse responded. "Our time has come to an end. At this place, while you did not see a new country or culture, you saw the things that go on behind closed doors of another girl just around your age. You saw the privileges that so many children take for granted, the challenges that burden children like Janie, and how we are all similar in the way we seek guidance in life and find joy in the daily things. From these last three nights with me, you have learned many things to carry forward into daily life. It's time for us to go now."

All at once, Millie was tossed through the darkness and the swirling colors; then, her body was met by the thump she had come to recognize. When she opened her eyes, she was surprised to find them wet with tears. Her heartfelt, both full and heavy, as she considered all the things other people worldwide and in her city experienced. Their lives were so different, yet; they were much more similar than she had ever realized. The pale moonlight shone through her white canopy, and she fell asleep thinking of all the things human beings have in common. "Tomorrow, I'm going to make friends with Claudia. I'm going to hear her story," Millie said to herself as she drifted back off to sleep beneath the light of the Moon.

The Prince and the Garden

Part 1: Princely Duties

"Amani," a husky voice cut through the blue-light of the dawn before the sun had risen. The voice was enough to command even the darkness. Prince Amani shot up from his pillow at the sound of it, rubbing the sleep to his cheeks, marked by the depth of his sleep. In the doorway stood an unmistakable booming figure—the kind which could only exist if given the space to. It was the Prince's father, King Julius. The Prince watched his father twist the wiry hairs of his beard around his stealthy fingers, in the way he often did while distressed or deep in thought.

"My son," the King spoke, "I am disheartened. Why do you still slumber when you know the pasture awaits your tenacity. The face of a King must shine even before the face of the sun has risen upon his kingdom. To command the rest of the world, you must have the fortitude to rise from your bed before it." "I'm sorry, Papa," the Prince stammered, jumping from his bed in search of his riding gear.

The King solemnly shook his head. "I don't know what it is that keeps you awake into the hours of the night from which no good thing has ever come. But you have duties to attend to. Becoming King is a task that takes your vigilance in every moment. Do not let this happen again." "Yes, papa," the Prince responded, refusing to meet the eyes of his father. Their eyes were the same shade of chestnut brown, but there was stoniness to the King's eyes that could make even the bravest shoulders cower.

Prince Amani rushed about the room, hurriedly pulling on his olive-green tunic and leather boots. His hair extended in hickory wisps of curls in all directions, and he made only a half-hearted attempt to tame them with a splash of water from the granite washtub. His heart pounded as he tried to ready himself in less than two minutes. The King did not like to wait.

The Prince bolted out of the oaken double doors of his bedroom and dashed down the corridor, nearly slipping on the freshly polished marble. At the end of the corridor was a winding staircase, which the Prince jumped down three at a time. He reached the bottom and bolted through the maze of corridors leading to the Far West End of the palace door. This was the door that led to the pasture.

He slowed his pace a bit as he began to walk through the grass, the morning dew slickening the leather on his boots. He made his way to the looming stable. "Sahil!" The Prince bellowed, "I am ready for my horse." Sahil was a boy about the Prince's age, with a long braid course and fair as the horse's hair themselves. He wore a tunic that was stained with mud and too small around the shoulders. The Prince watched him round the corner hurriedly, holding the end of a long rope. Attached to the other end of the rope was Prince Amani's valiant Arabian horse, glimmering white in the blue-black dawn. "Good morning, Persia," the Prince whispered, breath taken at the sight of his steed.

Sahil helped the Prince to situate his fine leather saddle on Persia's back. He climbed on and off they went into the pasture. The early morning's breeze was cool against the Prince's cheeks, blowing his hickory curls in more directions. He searched the field far and wide, wondering where his father could be.

Suddenly, the Prince heard a voice cutting through the darkness and felt struck from the back. Persia let out a startled whinny and reared her front legs in defense. Holding on tightly to the saddle horn, the Prince turned over his shoulder to face his attacker. Fixed there behind him was the King, upon his Black Stallion, wielding a sword that cut like a knife through the sheet of morning mist. "A noble king must always be prepared for the unexpected," his father said.

The Prince brought his hand to the side of his tunic, only to realize that he had forgotten to retrieve his sword before leaving the bedroom. "Papa, I've forgotten my sword upstairs," he said. The Prince was glad he could not see his father's face clearly through the mist, as he knew that all he would find there was a stone-cold disappointment.

"My son, I have no words for this," the King said with a sigh. "Come, let's gallop. You must keep Persia in top condition, for you never know when you will need her to run like the wind. She must learn the stealth and power that is required of a King's horse."

The King set off into the mist at top speed, leaving the Prince and Persia in his wake. "Hee-yah! Let's go, girl!" Prince Amani exclaimed, driving the heals of his leather boots into Persia's pearly hides. She began to gallop, and once again, the Prince felt the cool of the morning rustling his hair with the thrill of an entire day ahead. He drove his heels into Persia's hides again, and once more until she was running so fast, the Prince was sure at any moment they might leave the ground.

They sprinted through the pasture until the grass turned to sand. The Prince had reached the beach. His father was farther down the shore, his victorious figure silhouetted against the sea rocks. The Prince galloped up to his father, taking notice of the way his father glanced out upon the vastness of the sea with confidence and pride.

"Amani, my son," the King spoke, "this is our land."

"But Papa," Amani stammered, "how can humans own the sea? Especially when we have no idea what lies beneath it, or across it even a few thousand miles?" The King's gaze did not shift. "We own the sea because we own everything within our sight. This is what it means to be royalty. "Although the Prince still had questions, he chose instead to focus his gaze on the rhythmic crashing of the waves against the shore. The sun would soon rise, transforming the mist of dawn to a drizzle of glimmering gold before evaporating into the morning.

The King spoke again, "Tomorrow, you will wake up half an hour earlier, and you will not forget your sword. I must begin to see greater persistence in you, my son. I must begin to see you awaken ready to make the world your own."

"Of course, Papa," the Prince whispered. His voice got lost in the crash of the waves.

***

"Young Prince! Young Prince, awake, your breakfast is served."

Prince Amani blinked his long, dark lashes once, twice, and a third time as the blurred image of a shadowy figure holding a tray begin to materialize. He shook himself awake, stunned to see that he had fallen asleep in the desk chair in the corner of the room where he had been instructed to write the sentence "I will take ownership of the day and all that I encounter," five hundred times in calligraphy before breakfast.

"What is it today, Karmel?" the Prince asked.

"Blueberry hibiscus hotcakes, eggs benedict, and green tea mango matcha," Karmel answered. He had already left the bedside to busy himself opening the Prince's cashmere curtains.

"Delicious!" Amani exclaimed. "Tell me, Karmel, have you eaten?"

Amani watched the waiter sink into himself, refusing to meet Amani's eyes. "I am fine, Young Prince," Karmel said shyly.

"I did not ask if you were fine," Amani said pointedly, "I asked if you had eaten. Please, Karmel, sit with me. I can't eat all of these blueberry hibiscus hotcakes on my own."

Karmel glanced sheepishly at the steaming plate, piled ten cakes high. He certainly was hungry. But palace servants sharing a meal with royalty was strictly forbidden.

"I- I can't," Karmel responded.

Prince Amani felt his heart sink in guilt and dismay. He knew the palace rules, but he could not understand why they were what they were. "Karmel," he spoke gently, "come here." Prince Amani retrieved four blueberry hibiscus hot cakes from the top of the stack and tenderly wrapped them in a linen napkin. "For if you get hungry later," he said with a wink.

Karmel gingerly tucked the linen napkin in the side pocket of his tunic, making sure to fold in all the edges to it would stay put and not be seen. He bowed curtly to the Prince, and the Prince responded by placing his hands at his heart and bowing gently back. "Have a blessed day, my friend," Prince Amani said.

***

Prince Amani sat in the desk chair, staring out his True Arc windows to a lush landscape, rolling hills, the vast blue sea glistening in the morning brightness, and red roofs of the village houses below. From his tenth-story window in the palace, the village looked like a painting. The Prince sighed, thinking of how little he knew of this kingdom he was the heir to. What were the lives of the villagers like? The only villagers the Prince knew were Karmel, who came to work as servants in the palace. The royalty was expected not to interact more than necessary with their servants, and they were forbidden from given the servants access to any of the palace leisures.

Any reports of going against this ruling could have the servants cast out from their jobs. Prince Amani had tried many times to ask his father why these rules existed, to which his father only replied, "We must ensure that everyone stays in their rightful place." This never made sense to the Prince, but he had learned that his father's arguments were seldom won.

Although Prince Amani often tried to befriend the palace servants, they were very hesitant about his friendship. They needed to keep their jobs to survive and provide for their families. Although being a servant at the castle provided very little, it was enough for daily bread and a weekly broth pot.

The Prince was suddenly jarred from his daydreaming by the sound of his heavy oaken doors thrown open. In ambled Poppy, a spritely young girl from the village was always bursting with passion, enthusiasm, and quick-witted responses. Poppy reminded the Prince of a flickering flame, who could set the world ablaze with her passion if only given the opportunity. She dreamt of being a poet, but those dreams were put aside to serve as the message bearer for the royal family by day and care for her sickly mother each evening. She had come this morning to deliver the Prince's agenda for the day.

"Good morning, Young Prince!" Poppy bellowed, "I come bearing your daily schedule. Another sunrise, another day of princely duties!"

Prince Amani settled against the back of the chair, waiting expectantly for Poppy to begin her recitation.

10:00 a.m: Strength training in the palace gym

11:00 a.m: Bathe and dress for a successful day

11:30 a.m: Recitation practice

1:00 p.m: Lunch in the Great Hall

2:00 p.m: Afternoon tea with Princess Potentials

4:00 p.m: Reading and calligraphy annotation of "The Keeping of a Kingdom."

6:30 p.m: Dinner in the Great Hall

8:00 p.m: Orchestra viewing in the foyer

9:00 p.m: Bedtime routine

"Thank you, Poppy," the Prince said.

"Certainly, Young Prince. Now, you'd best hurry and fetch your gym clothes," she replied.

Part 2: To Be King

"Young Prince, a King does not begin his recitation with slumped shoulders. You must command the space with your body before you even begin to speak," directed Prince Amani's recitation coach, Lizette. Lizette was the best in the kingdom when it came to grammar, diction, and speaking skills. She had been the recitation coach for so long that she had earned a place living in the palace basement, marking her with a higher status than many of the other servants. Lizette was well-respected, and she worked to make the Bradbury Palace's recitations the best in all the land.

The Prince was doing his echo-exercises, in which he had to say the phrase: "Good afternoon, the kingdom of Bradbury" with enough strength to make it echo back to him from across the room. "To deliver your message well, your voice must travel with a purpose. You must project your voice from your diaphragm to the wall across this room. Allow your voice to hit the opposite wall and bounce back with a force and sharpness strong enough to pierce a man's heart," Lizette commanded.

Each time the Prince spoke, Lizette stopped him in his tracks and demanded he begins again. When it was not the volume of his voice, she critiqued, it was the way he held his body. After nearly an hour of this routine, Prince Amani began to feel his face fall with exhaustion. "Young Prince," Lizette's voice cut through his daze, "if a King cannot maintain a face of energy and vigilance, how shall he earn the respect of his kingdom? How shall he respect anyone to bow before him, to take his word as the utmost truth?"

The Prince wanted to say that he believed no person in the land held the utmost truth, but he did not. Instead, he straightened his shoulders, blinking his eyes a few times in the attempt to revive himself. He began to speak again. "Good afternoon, Bradbury... kingdom... of... my kingdom... Bradbury," his words escaped him. The Prince could not control himself; he felt the corners of his mouth begin to curve upwards in a grin. Lizette tapped her foot impatiently. "A king must maintain a straight face, no matter the circumstances. You must not allow anything to derail you during a recitation. Begin again." With a sigh, the Prince began his introduction again, and again, and again. By the time the recitation practice was over, the Prince had still not heard his voice bounce back to him off the opposite wall with the force and sharpness to pierce a chest. Why would a king want to pierce the chests of his followers anyway?

***

Several hours later, the Prince stared at his reflection in one of the Grande Mirrors of the corridor. He half-heartedly attempted to calm his hickory curls and spread his lips to ensure that none of the kale salad from lunch had wedged itself between his teeth.

It was time for afternoon tea.

Several afternoons a week, royal girls would come to the palace from other kingdoms to have tea with the Prince. He was meant to evaluate each one until he found one he might like to marry. On some occasions, village girls would be invited to the teas as well, granted that Miriam the Matchmaker saw them fit to sit at the same table as the Prince. It was supposed to be a great honor for a girl to be invited to a tea with the Prince, although he could never understand what made him so special. Each of the girls he met was just fine on their own, and he believed there was much more to each of them than how she would serve as a wife or Queen.

At every tea, Prince Amani was given a sheet of paper with each young woman's name. He was to begin by ranking her beauty on a scale of 1-10. The Prince could not bring himself to do this because he saw every girl who sat in front of him as beautiful. Instead, he preferred to write the qualities he loved most about each of the girls next to their names. Today there were three Princess Potentials.

There was Princess Lillian, a princess of chocolate eyes and auburn hair wearing a dress the shade of lilacs. Princess Lillian came from the nearby kingdom of Ballannon. Then there was Princess Jade of the domain of Borendale, whose eyes matched her name and whose hair flowed down her back like ebony satin. Princess Jade wore a dress in a shade of scarlet that burned like the ring around the sun when it rose. If either Princess were to be chosen, she would leave her kingdom and her family and move into the Bradbury Palace. Prince Amani did not think it was fair that a princess should have to leave everything she had known her entire life only to come to be the Queen to a man of another kingdom and another family. Every Princess he had met was capable of adopting a kingdom herself, without the help of anyone. He had once asked his father if he chose a princess as his Queen if he could move to her kingdom, instead of expecting her to move to his. To this, his father replied, "Absolutely not. That is just not the way it is done."

The third Princess Potential was a village girl named Lorelei, with olive skin and piercing eyes the sea's color. Lorelei was one of the village girls deemed fit to bring Miriam, the Matchmaker, to bring to the palace. She was the daughter of a baker. Lorelei wore a simple dress in a light blue shade that made her eyes shine even bluer.

The Prince had also asked his father once what would be done if a village girl was chosen and did not want to leave her village. What if she wanted to stay with her family or follow her dreams in the town? To this, the King responded, "My son, these questions show me that you have no understanding of how the world works. Any woman would be glad to rise above the place she has been born into; marrying into royalty is the only way for her and her family to have a better life."

Miriam, the Matchmaker, sat close to the Prince, sipping her tea nervously. At every tea, he was given a list of questions he was supposed to ask the girls. However, the Prince often liked to stray from the list and engage with the young women in ways that were not written. It was in this way that he came to understand the young women better as people. Prince Amani glanced at the first question on the list. "What are the manners a Queen must adapt to the table?"

Princess Lillian raised her hand to speak and waited for the Prince to call on her. "A Queen must not talk at the table unless she is spoken to. She must sit with grace and poise, with her napkin in her lap, repeatedly dabbing at her mouth to ensure nothing gets left behind. When she drinks from a chalice or a teacup with a handle, she must raise her pinky daintily, and she must be careful not to make any noise with her dishes or silverware.

She must chew each bite of food exactly thirty-seven times before swallowing. Lastly, she shall not rise from the table until the King has moved his seat back."

Prince Amani fidgeted in discomfort. While this was the answer written on the sheet, it was not one he agreed with. Miriam kicked the Prince under the table, nudging him to tell the Princess she had answered correctly. When the Prince didn't respond, Miriam cleared her throat. "That's correct, Lillian," she said.

"Next question," said the Prince, "Which material is better for a gown, silk or chiffon?" Lorelei shifted in her seat, keeping her piercing blue eyes narrowed on her tea. Princess Jade raised her hand. "Chiffon is well-suited for a typical day, but the most upscale evening gowns should always be silk." The Prince nodded, "That's correct, Princess," he said.

Instead of moving on to the third question, the Prince set down the sheet. "Now, I want to know something about each of you. What is the thing that makes your soul sing?" He watched confusion fall over Jade and Lillian's faces like a heavy fog. Lorelei's eyes, however, shot up from her tea glass. She raised her hand. "Yes, Lorelei?" the Prince said with a grin. "The thing that makes my soul sing most is playing the piano. My mother taught me to play when I was young. When I was ten, there was a fire in my father's old bakery, the one we lived above. My mother was killed. We lost everything, and my father had to rebuild the bakery on the roadside. There is no piano there, so I play the one in the old church when I can. I hardly have time because I am so busy caring for my younger sister and two younger brothers. But my biggest dream is to be a pianist, traveling to all the kingdoms in the land, playing in palaces like this. I would rebuild my father's bakery and a nice cottage for the family with the money I made..." she trailed off.

Jade raised her hand. "The dream that makes my heart sing is to be a painter. I love to do portraits, and I wish I could spend all day in the village, painting portraits of the villagers I see." Then Lillian spoke. "The dream that makes my heart sing is to take over my father's kingdom for myself. I have learned everything there is to know about running a kingdom. I wake up every morning before the sun and ride my horse; we are strong and well-trained. I am a talented writer, and I speak with a spirited voice. I only wish my voice could be heard." The Prince thought hard about what each young woman had said. They wished to use their passions and skills to lift themselves. They did not need a King to do it for them. Prince Amani did not speak. He took his pen and wrote next to each girl's name.

Lillian: "Fiery and independent. When she speaks, she commands. The world listens. She is wise and fearless and cannot be derailed. She should have a kingdom of her own."

Jade: "Creative and compassionate. Wishes to paint people for who they are. She longs to be free to roam."

Lorelei: "Caring and dedicated to her family. She is a pianist who dreams of using her passion for lifting the ones she loves most. She is not derailed by the odds being set against her; she knows how to persist."

The Prince continued to sit quietly, studying his notes. Miriam looked at him expectantly. "Thank you, princesses, for joining me for tea today. I have loved the opportunity to know what makes your hearts sing. I regret to inform you, however, that I am feeling ill from lunch. I think I should retire to my room for a bit. Feel free to stay and chat as long as you like; Miriam will fetch you whatever you need. And Lorelei, there's a piano in the foyer that you're welcome to," the Prince said. Before Miriam could stop him, he pushed his chair back from the table and bolted up the winding marble staircase, down the corridor, and through the oaken doors to his room.

Part 3: A Gardener's Wisdom

That afternoon, the Prince was meant to be annotating "The Keeping of a Kingdom." His father called this book "The King's Bible," saying it had all the information necessary to become a successful King. However, Prince Amani was coming to understand that his idea of success was quite different from his father's. The Prince's idea of a prosperous kingdom was one where every villager felt seen and understood. Why were there people like him, living in palaces so big someone could get lost, when people in the village below were forced to have their businesses along the road and share one loaf of bread between the family and a pot of bone broth each week, if they were lucky? Why did they have the most luxurious teas and biscuits in all the land in the Palace when villagers were going to sleep hungry? Why was the only way a woman could be a success was if a successful human-made her so?

Prince Amani closed the book before he had even gotten through the first page. There was only one person with whom he could speak on instances such as these. Hastily, the Prince began to make his way across the floor to the oaken doors. He pushed the door open quietly, checking both directions of the corridor to ensure it was clear. He could not be seen by anyone, especially not by anyone who might tell his father he had been wandering. After seeing the coast was clear, the Prince turned the opposite direction of the winding staircase. He shuffled down the hallway to a door at the very end, which opened to a secret staircase.

This staircase led down and out into the palace gardens. When he arrived in the gardens, the Prince began to search among the daffodils, tulips, lavender, hibiscus, and Queen Anne's Lace. After a few moments, he heard the familiar sound of whistling. He trotted along the garden path until he saw a faded brown suede hat bobbing above the rosebushes. A man lifted his head and found the Prince with a smile. The corners of the man's eyes were crinkled with kindness, and his face was weathered smooth and copper from many days under the sun.

"Angelo!" The Prince exclaimed, "I am so happy to see you, my friend."

"What are you sneaking away from this afternoon, my friend?" Angelo asked with a twinkle in his eye.

"Oh, Angelo, it was awful. I overslept again this morning and woke up to my father's disappointment in me. Once I got out on the pasture, I realized I had forgotten to equip myself with my sword. During my recitation practice, I couldn't even get past the introduction without being reprimanded for the way I held my body, the way my voice hit the wall or the way I couldn't keep a straight face. After lunch, I had another afternoon tea with Potential Princesses, and all I could think was how guilty I felt that these young women had to come to me for their future when their future already lies within them. I cannot pick a princess to become my Queen one day, not because they are not all beautiful and worthy of love, but because each of them has hopes and dreams that would be better off without me, without this Palace, and without the way of the kingdom. My father tells me this is 'just how things are,' but I wonder, is there no room for change? Everything I am taught to be strength comes only by force. Is force truly the best way?"

"My friend," Angelo spoke, "take a lesson from the tending of the garden. The flowers know how to grow on their own. When the winds of change shake their stems and leaves, they tuck inside themselves and hold firm in their roots until the storm has passed. When it is Time for new growth, they shed their withered leaves to make room for the new. It is the gardener's job to be aware of his flower's needs and prepare himself to aid them when he can. When it has been a while since the rain has fallen, I gather water myself to pour into the flowers and nourish them. When they need a little help shedding their old leaves and petals to make room for the new, I will tend to them with gentle hands. The rest of my job is to watch, to wait, and to speak kindly to.

Everything grows better with kindness. My strength is in gentleness with which I tend the flowers, the faith I put in their ability to grow, the divinity I see in them, and the space I give them for their journey." The Prince nodded thoughtfully, trying to make sure he understood everything Angelo was saying.

"These young women you have met, they are like flowers. Capable of their brilliance, their growth. Everyone benefits from being nourished and poured into, but the most important thing is to hold space. Each of these young women has her dream, her purpose. The way to address them is with a gentle spirit that recognizes the divinity in each of them as she is with or without a prince at her side. I believe that you have seen this," Angelo said.

"But Angelo," the Prince spoke, "what am I to do in a place that does not see strength in gentleness or in holding space for the journey of others?" A shadow of contemplation fell across Angelo's face. "My friend, it is not easy in a world whose expectations are meant to keep you growing only in one direction. Like the flowers change positions to turn their faces to the sun, so you must turn your face in the direction of your growth. It will not be easy. You will always have hands grabbing at you, telling you, 'No, not that way.' But only you can determine your proper direction. You must follow your own sun."

Angelo was always so poetic in the way he spoke. Although Prince Amani enjoyed it, sometimes he grew tired and needed a break. "Angelo, will you tell me about the creatures of the garden?" the Prince asked. Each day he stole away from his princely duties to meet Angelo in the garden; he was met by explanations of another plant or animal species. To the Prince, Angelo was perhaps the wisest man in the world.

"Ah, yes," Angelo said with a twinkle in his eye, "Come, let me show my Cattleya Orchid friends." He led Angelo down the path to a cluster of flowers in various shades of pastel purple, honey-yellow, and violet. Each Cattleya Orchid looked as if she had her eyes closed restfully, and her mouth poised to begin a song at any moment. "My cattleyas represent love and beauty," said Angelo, "my friend, you should know that love is at the core of every human. Love itself is the reason we are here. Love is all there truly is."

The Prince pondered this as they began to continue down the garden path. Just near the garden pond, Angelo stopped before they were rows and rows of flowers blushing light pink and magenta, with deep red spots that looked like freckles. "These are the Stargazer Lilies," Angelo spoke, "The pink shades symbolize abundance and prosperity. There is something you should know about prosperity, as there are many misconceptions. While many people think it is represented in palaces like your own, of marble floors, exotic meals, grand pianos, silk gowns, servants, fine wine, and even luscious gardens such as this, it is something far greater than this. True prosperity is within the heart. A man will only ever be as rich as he is rooted in the small joys and gratitudes of his own life and his essence."

The two continued to stroll down the path to the other side of the garden pond. The Prince took notice of the koi fish in the pond, gliding back and forth in hues of gold, cream, and fiery orange. He wondered what it might be like to be a fish with no expectation but to swim. As if reading his mind, Angelo stopped at the pond and began to focus on the ripples of the fish gliding by. "The koi fish symbolizes good fortune and perseverance through adversity. They represent the courage and persistence required to advance along the stream of life to be reborn. Just as the fish persists in swimming even when the waters are rough, so we must persist towards the destination of our most true selves."

After the two sat and meditated on the koi fish's movement beneath the rippling pond waters, they continued towards the East Wall of the garden. Angelo stopped again just ahead of one side of the stone wall, which enclosed the gardens. At the foot of the wall, there was a bush of waxy white flowers enveloped in leaves of polished green. The fragrance hit the Prince's nostrils and made his body feel light with bliss. He closed his eyes and breathed the fragrance deep into his lungs, feeling its euphoria coarse through his entire being. "This," whispered Angelo, "is the gardenia. The flower of a gentle spirit. As the power of this aroma over your body, so too is the power of a gentle spirit in moving in the world."

At that moment, the Prince that dusk was beginning to fall on the garden. The sky was fading to pink, orange, and lilac, which would soon give way to the blueish black hues of the moments in between day and night. The Prince felt his heart quicken, wondering if he might be late for dinner. Whenever he was in the garden with Angelo, it was as though Time did not exist. Every moment seemed to melt away.

"Angelo, I think I need to get back to the Palace. I may have missed dinner," the Prince said. "Thank you so much for sharing your wisdom with me; I hope to return to the garden soon."

"Rest well, my friend," Angelo said, his eyes once again crinkling in a gentle grin.

Prince Amani turned away, bounding down the garden path. He felt a melancholy sitting deep in his stomach, the same one he always felt when it came to leaving the garden. When he went to the garden, every worry melted away with the passing moments, and he thought he could be genuinely himself. He learned more from the garden and Angelo than he had ever learned in his Princely Lessons.

***

As one day unfolded into the next, Prince Amani stole away to the garden whenever he could get the chance. Sometimes, he awoke in the middle of the night and spent Time beneath the moonlight, walking or sitting among his flower friends and letting their wisdom wash over them. Simply spending Time alongside the flowers made the Prince's own heart spread open like petals to the sun.

When Angelo was there during the day, he introduced the Prince to new gardening techniques and taught him about every creature's essence in the garden. The Prince learned that the soil where the flowers' roots were embedded was just as much alive as the flowers themselves. He showed the Prince how the scraps of food from the kitchen could be composted to feed the soil and nourish it. In terms of light, every species of flower needed a different amount of light, and some even required shade. Angelo had sown the garden seeds intentionally in places where he knew the sun would nourish them in just the right way. The Prince was taught how to tell when there would be rain that day by how heavy the air felt upon his skin or if he saw a ring around the moon in the evening. "Water is a lifegiving force," Angelo said, "but too much of anything is enough to drown out the life. It is with great caution that we must water the garden."

The two became good friends. Often, Prince Amani was the one who talked about his life problems and asked Angelo for advice. The Prince often wondered how a man came to know so much about the universe, as Angelo did. Angelo was always willing to listen and offer advice where it was needed, but rarely did he speak about his own life. The Prince knew Angelo lived alone in the village, without a wife or any children. He had learned to garden at a young age when his mother harvested wildflower seeds and showed him how to sew them around the village. His horticultural skills had led him to his job at the Palace. The Prince also knew that Angelo walked to work each day, and his heels were callused from the miles which had weakened the soles of his sandals. The Prince resolved that one day, he would learn more about his friend.

***

Finally, the "one day" the Prince had dreamt of arrived. His parents were leaving Bradbury to travel to another kingdom, and he had begged them to allow him to stay home to study and practice his sword fighting maneuvers. This would be the day the Prince would ask Angelo to let him into the village with him to learn more of his life. After tea that afternoon, Angelo went up to his room, telling his servants he felt ill and not to worry about him for dinner.

The Prince bounded down the garden path, searching for his friend. Once again, he saw the brown suede hat bobbing above the rosebushes. "Angelo, hello!" the Prince chimed. "Hello, my friend," Angelo greeted him. "Angelo, for all these days, you have poured your wisdom on me like water in the garden. You have nourished me and taught me how the garden could be a space to find peace and feel seen. You have given me a listening ear, inspired the courage to grow in my own direction, and held space for me. Now, I want to know more about your life. May I come with you to the village tonight?"

"My friend," Angelo spoke with concern, "it is hazardous for you to leave the palace grounds. Not only this, but I have very little to offer you in my home."

"Angelo, please let me join you. You are my friend, and I want to share this experience with you," the Prince said. Angelo cast a glance over each shoulder as if checking to see if the coast was clear. He let out his breath and turned to face the Prince. "Okay," he said, "but we must try to keep you out of sight. If anyone from the Palace finds out you are gone, we will both be in grave trouble."

With that, the two set off through the gate and beyond the stone walls surrounding the garden. The Prince noticed the sun's radiance on the sea, making the waves like jewels in the moments between the light and dark. He noticed a slight ache in his feet, but he did not speak upon it. His boots were indeed sturdier than the worn sandals Angelo wore on this trekking day in and day out.

The road began to slope as they started their descent to the village. The terrain was rocky and surrounded by bristled grass. Although Angelo's frame was thinning with age and his hair turning gray and wiry, he was steadier on his feet than Prince Amani was as they navigated the slope. The Prince watched in awe as Angelo braced his body against the invisible force of gravity, moving swiftly, smoothly, and with ease. The Prince wondered to himself what it would be like to be so present, steadfast, and aware of one's role in the universe in the way Angelo was.

***

By the time they reached the village, night had already fallen. The last Time Prince Amani had been in the village was when he was very young for a recitation his father gave. They had traveled down the slope by carriage, and he had not looked upon the village streets in the way he did now. As darkness engulfed the village, Prince Amani noticed how many villagers did not have a home to return to. There were alleyways between buildings lined with makeshift shelters of boards, scrap metal, and cardboard and beds of tattered cloths on the ground. He saw a woman balancing a baby on her hip in one corner, boiling a pot of water over a stove fashioned out of heated stones. She pulled the pot off of the hot stones and retrieved a small bag of sugar and a spoon from the pocket of her frayed apron. He watched as the woman gingerly stirred four teaspoons of sugar into the boiling water.

She turned to two children, a boy and a girl; their slight frames bent together in the corner. The woman spooned the boiled sugar water into the mouth of the girl first, then the boy. After this, she tried to slip some of the water between the baby's lips. The woman took none of the water for herself. "Angelo," the PrincePrince whispered, "haven't they got more to eat than this?" Angelo shook his head, solemnly. "My friend, only the luckiest of us get the weekly bread and broth. Many people in this village eat no more some days than boiled sugar water or nothing at all."

The Prince was stunned. "What do the villagers without homes do when the winter strikes? The winters here are so bitter cold." Angelo could not meet the Prince's eyes. "Villagers without homes make stone stoves and try to warm themselves with each other's bodies. Many of them do not survive the winter. Those of us who are fortunate enough to have shelter try to open our doors to those who do not, but it is impossible to have enough food or blankets for everyone. And when some of us fall ill, it becomes a scary time for all."

The Prince could say nothing in return. He felt a horrible gnawing in his stomach which made him no longer feel hungry for the dinner he had missed that evening. The houses lining the streets where villagers did live were weathered and worn, with broken windows, hanging wires, and many windowsills lit only by a candle. And yet, even from the street, the Prince could hear the sounds of life behind thin walls. He heard singing, laughter, and prayers of gratitude for the day. As if reading his mind, Angelo said, "Yes, my friend. Even with so little, we still are blessed. Gratitude does more to feed our souls than bread or broth. It is the act of being thankful for what we have that fuels us and keeps us moving from one day to the next. As long as humans have love, and someone to keep them company, to find a home in, to consider family, we can persist through life's daily difficulties. We can feed one another's souls."

His thoughts were soon interrupted when Angelo spoke up again, "We're here."

In front of them sat a small hut fashioned out of mud bricks. The cookstove was located outside the house, a little bit of stones with a pot hanging above; it was just as the woman in the alley had. Angelo pushed open a rounded door with stargazer lilies painted on it.

"Did you paint this?" The Prince asked. "Yes," said Angelo, "using pressed mulberries, violets, and particles of light pink seashells from the beach. I wanted to remind myself each time I come home of the abundance in my life."

Inside the house was a small room containing only a sleeping mat and a wooden board fashioned into a table with half a loaf of bread, a knife, a candle, and a bones pile.

"The bones are gathered from behind the butcher shop. Meat is a delicacy many villagers cannot afford, so we boil the bones in water to make broth. I wish I could have a vegetable garden in which to grow carrots and potatoes and perhaps some other vegetables to put with my broth, but the soil in the village is too dry and not compact enough for anything to grow."

Prince Amani watched as Angelo gathered the bones up from the wooden board, then placed them in the pot. "I already fetched the water this morning," Angelo said, "there is only one well in town for public use, and I usually go before the sun rises."

Angelo rubbed two sticks together to light the candle, then held it to heat the stones. Once the water was boiling, he went back inside to fetch the bread and the knife.

He split the loaf into two small pieces. "Isn't this your last loaf? Please, don't worry about me. I'll be fine," the Prince said. "That is not how it works," said Angelo, "you are a guest in my home, and whatever I have, you must also have."

"Angelo," the Prince said, "who do you have? Who feeds your soul?"

"I once had a woman who was a piece of my soul in the flesh. Everything missing in me was in her. I had never known home until I saw her eyes," his eyes grew far away as he spoke, "In her womb grew a child out of the seeds of our love. I lost them both one winter to a fever. My grief made me wish the fever had taken me too. But over time, I healed and was led back to the importance of love. Love is the only thing that truly matters, and I had to cultivate it in my life again. Gardening has given me that opportunity. I sowed the seeds of something new and waited patiently, nourishing them to grow. When I tend to the flowers and observe the creatures, learning from them and nourishing them is love. Just as I tend to the garden, I try to tend to the needs of other villagers. Anyone who knocks at my door in search of bread or a roof above their head for a night can share mine. I have little, but what I have can always be shared with someone who has less. Love is what feeds my soul, and it takes many forms."

Part 4: A King's Calling

After sharing a meal of bread and bone broth with Angelo, the Prince prepared himself to go back up the slope to the Palace. "My friend, that is not safe. The slope is dangerous to navigate in the dark. There are wild animals about at night, not to mention the village thieves. Thieves are the only people who have had their needs unmet for too long.

But still, you could be hurt."

Prince Amani scratched his head, attempting to think of a solution. "You will sleep here tonight. At dawn, you will wake and make your way back up the slope. Be sure to stay out of sight in the village to avoid causing a spectacle. If your father sees you approaching, you will tell him you chose to go for a strengthening walk before sun up. You must not be suspicious in any way."

The Prince watched as Angelo removed a threadbare blanket from the top of his sleeping mat and spread it on the ground next to the mat. "You will have the mat tonight," Angelo said, "and I will have the blanket. This makes a place for both of us to lay our heads." The Prince did not try to argue, as he knew at this point that any argument he posed would not be won. He took his place upon Angelo's sleeping mat, and the two lay together in the dark. "Thank you for bringing me here, Angelo, and for telling me your story," the Prince said. "My friend, thank you for coming here and for asking me," Angelo replied.

Angelo was off to sleep quickly after this, but The Prince tossed and turned all night, unable to get a wink of sleep. His mind was whirring with everything he had just seen. Nothing in him could understand how some people in the kingdom could have so little while he and his family enjoyed so much. And even so, he did not laugh with his parents how he heard the laughter of the villagers echo from behind thin walls. There was no singing, no prayers, no gratitudes. And even though his parents had access to all the riches in the land, they had no generosity in their spirits to bless others.

"I cannot be King of a kingdom where we cannot share in each other's joys and abundances. I cannot be King of a kingdom where people die of the winter or where mothers feed their children boiled water with rationed sugar. I cannot be King of a kingdom where love is not the entirety." The Prince thought of what Angelo had said about the desire to grow food in a vegetable garden. The soil in the village was not fit for gardening, but Angelo knew the Palace's soil was. The palace soil had been toiled and cultured until it offered enough nutrients to grow hundreds of species of flowers. If flowers could grow there, perhaps other things could as well. Perhaps there was more to running a kingdom than he had ever known before. Maybe it was not what Amani could receive from running a kingdom—the riches, the horses, the silk sheets, the servants, the exotic foods and teas—perhaps it was, instead, what could be given and what could grow.

***

When Angelo woke with the onset of dawn, he found the Prince already awake and staring up at the ceiling. "Did you get any sleep?" Angelo asked the Prince.

Prince Amani grinned. "No, but I had plenty of dreams." With that, the Prince stood up, thanked his friend, and began his journey back through the village and up the slope towards the Palace. He ducked behind corners and glanced over his shoulders to make sure no one had caught sight of him. Amani had come to understand that the greatest strength of all was to risk being seen in all that he stood for. No longer would he stay silent. No longer would he allow himself to be concealed in the world of having everything and yet still wanting more that laid beyond the thick palace walls.

The Prince became so distracted by the sound of his thoughts that the trek up the slope seemed nearly easy. His heartbeat in anticipation and he could not be sure if what he felt was fear or invincibility. Perhaps it was both. Whatever this feeling in his heart was, it felt like truth. Amani stopped for a moment to catch his breath, looking out at the sun rising like a ball of fire in a rose gold world. As he breathed the cold weight of the morning into his nostrils, feeling it settle around his lungs, he thought of how the painting looked much less like a painting from where he now stood, beyond the True Arc window, beyond the palace walls.

Suddenly, Prince Amani was not merely looking upon the hills; he was rolling among them, feeling the precariousness of loose earth beneath his feet, with only sparing blades of grass to grab onto. The sea seemed less like something for faraway viewing pleasure, and more like something in which to immerse oneself, letting the sea teach any lessons it wished to a surrendered body, whose only choice was to swim with the currents. The red roofs of the village houses below were no longer faraway objects of a place Amani could not understand the feelings of. He had now slept beneath such a roof. He had walked the streets that wound beneath these houses, his feet becoming familiar with the soil in which nothing could grow. He had glanced through the broken windows at the unnamed bodies eating bread and broth, thinking of how he should know their names and how they should have more to eat than bread and broth. He had seen other bodies too, the bodies of those who had not even a red roof to seek shelter beneath, who cowered in the corners of the streets and shifted between wanting to be seen for being human and wanted to stay out of sight to feel still safe.

The feeling that came to Amani next began in the pit of his stomach and rose as a pang in his throat. He felt the weight of everything he had ever had the privilege to call his own, simply because of where he was born and who he was born to. He felt the weight of his silk sheets and the breakfast he so greatly hungered for after just one night of eating only bread and broth. He felt the weight of the grand piano and the dreams behind every pair of eyes he had glanced into over tea—dreams which always seemed to come second to the potential of royalty.

As the Prince approached the palace wall, he saw a vine snaking up the side. He pulled it to ensure it could support his weight, then hoisted himself up, scurrying up the side of the wall. He jumped, landing in the lush, dew-wet grass with a thud. The sun had almost turned from orange to the kind of yellow you could not look into without searing your eyes, which made Prince Amani think he must be late to meet his father. He decided to skip horse riding today and tell his father that he had simply gone for a walk in the garden. Today was the day the Prince began his journey towards the King he would be and the kingdom he would build.

***

For many days after this, the Prince stole away from the kingdom whenever he got the chance. Angelo taught the Prince everything there was to know about gardening. The Prince learned about the types of soil and which types were needed to nourish various crops. He asked Miriam to acquire as many fruit and vegetable seeds as she could in order to have organic produce. Miriam seemed perplexed, but she was not one to question orders.

Amani and Angelo determined a plot of land in which to plant and made plans to begin their work in the spring. Throughout the months that followed, the Prince spent the Time he was supposed to be studying his "princely duties" to reading books from the Palace library on species of vegetables, orchards, and grains that could be grown. Day after day, the Prince prayed that he would be shown how to extend care to the people of his kingdom so that one day when he inherited it, every life would feel cared for, supported, and loved.

Not only did the Prince engage in his gardening passion day in and out through the books he read and the conversations he had with Angelo, but he also made a point in his life to hear the stories and passions of the people he saw every day. He spoke to the servants and cooks of the Palace (even grumpy Miriam), asking them where they came from, what brought them joy, and what they dreamt of accomplishing in life.

When the princess prospects came to the Palace for tea, Amani asked them similar questions. He wanted to see them for who they were—women with dreams and passions. Although this was not the everyday discourse of a Palace tea, Miriam grew to accept it after some time, and she warmed up to sharing her own story as well. The Prince learned that Miriam loved horses and that she dreamt of having a horse of her own to care for and participate in horse races. Month after month, as Amani's plans for his garden grew, so did his relationship with everyone he came across at the Palace.

***

Eventually, spring came to pass, and Angelo and the Prince began the hard-daily work of tilling the soil, planting the seeds, and tending the crops. They planted raspberry and blueberry bushes, patches of strawberry and rhubarb, peach trees, and apple trees. They grew wheat, barley, oats, lentils, soybeans, and every kind of vegetable known to man. The Prince began to read books on food preservation to distribute food among villagers in cans for the winter months. The Prince and Angelo made a cart from the winter's leftover firewood, in which they would carry the bounty of crops down the slope to the village in the summertime.

When the summer came, the garden crops grew plentiful and ready to be eaten. One afternoon, Angelo and the Prince worked tirelessly into nightfall harvesting the crops and loading them into the wooden cart. When morning came, the Prince woke before the sun. He crept across the dew-wet grass to the stables. He saddled Persia and hitched her to the cart, and all at once, they began their descent down the side of the slope into the village below.

As the Prince approached the village entrance, he saw Angelo there, just as promised. The two men began hastily assembling the cart with the garden's bounty. On the front of the cart, Angelo painted the words "A Summer Feast: Free for All." Throughout the day, hundreds of villagers paid visits to the Prince and Angelo, filling their baskets and sacks until all the fruits, vegetables, and grains had been gathered. As he looked upon each villager's face, Amani was struck by what it means to show love to one another.

That evening at dinner, the Prince knew it was time to tell his family what he had been doing. He pushed his food back and forth on his plate, waiting for a lull in the conversation. Finally, his moment came. "My son," his father spoke, "you've hardly spoken all evening. What are you thinking of?" The Prince looked up sheepishly, then thought to himself, "This is my strength. I must speak of it as such." He swallowed and summoned the courage from somewhere deep within himself. "I have news to share with you all," the Prince spoke.

His father and mother waited with expectant eyes, and Miriam stood in the kitchen doorway, trying not to make it evident that she was also listening. "I will inherit this kingdom one day, and there are some things that I must address—some things which have troubled me for a very long time," the Prince spoke. "I cannot understand how we can proudly run a kingdom and ignore the lives of every human being there, viewing them as less than ourselves and not much caring how they end up. How can we sit high in this Palace with the finest of linens and silks, exotic foods, and more room than we could ever need, while there are people below whose names we don't know, whose stomachs are going empty, and who is sleeping behind broken windows, beneath caving roofs, or worse, on street corners? We have so much, and we feel entitled to keep it all for ourselves. Not only this, but we do not even speak to the people who spend every day in this Palace with us. We expect them to serve us and do not pay any mind to who they are, the lives they lead, the dreams they hold, or how we may be able to help them." The PrincePrince stopped speaking, watching his parents blink at him. "I know that one day soon, I will inherit this kingdom. I have spent my entire life learning what strength should look like; what I am told it means to be a king. But where is the talk of the strength that lies in helping others? Where is the talk in the strength that lies in doing what we can to benefit this entire kingdom instead of simply presiding over it? I will not be the kind of King who has no regard for anything but his gain and power. That legacy ends with me."

The Prince felt nervous, unsure of what his parents may say, so he quickly launched the next thought. "I have spent nearly the last year learning how to cultivate a garden. I was taught by the gardener, a good friend of mine, and the wisest man I have ever known. I built a cart from old firewood and took Persia down the slope to the village, where I gave the abundance of fruits, vegetables, and grains away to the villagers. I think it would be lovely if we could spare some of our bounties for Miriam to make cakes and pastries and provide some of our meat. We always have far too much. And I think we ought to go among the villagers and repair every broken window and every sinking roof. We ought to provide the villagers with supplies to build their beds and tables and to heat their homes in the winter. We ought to have clothes tailored and provide books for the schoolchildren and enough to eat to attend school. When people are sick, we must send our Palace doctors and nurses to tend to them with our ample medical resources. I vow to make this kingdom one where everyone's needs are met—one in which I spend time with the villagers, visit their businesses, and attend their festivals," the Prince said.

He took another breath. "Finally, I will not marry a woman simply because that is what is expected of her. All of the princess prospects I've met have their visions, their dreams, their passions. I could easily love any of them, and perhaps I will. But it will not be because either of us is forced out of our dreams for the sake of what is expected of us."

Amani's parents continued to blink at him, stunned speechless. "My son," the King finally spoke, "This is just not how things have ever been." "Father," said the Prince, "we cannot let the way things have always been hold us back from what can be."

***

After the night Prince Amani spoke his truth, the kingdom began to experience a shift. Slowly, his father began to honor his suggestions. Miriam baked loaves of bread, cakes, and pastries, the garden continued to flourish; village children were brought to the castle to play the piano and ride the horses. The walls to the garden were knocked down, and villagers could come in to walk or help with the growth of flowers and crops. Everything that was in the Palace so was below in the village. Homes were built, sicknesses were cured, festivals were celebrated as a community, and the food markets with crops from the garden continued. Angelo grew too old to continue gardening, but the Prince continued his work. Angelo often sat out in front of his house, sipping tea from the Palace and smiling at how his village had changed as a result of the change of heart.

The kingdom continued to grow, and no one ever went sick, hungry, cold, or without school again. Children followed their dreams and learned that here, they could become whatever they aspired to be. Each night, when Prince Amani looked out upon the painting-like village below, he felt his heartbeat in anticipation of what his kingdom was becoming. Like the Palace garden below, Prince Amani's empire had grown abundant with care and gentle tending.

The Wisdom Tree

In every corner of the world, there are secrets that only the children know. The eyes of adults are trained in what to see, and they often miss the magic in daily life. In some places, there are trees who have been rooted in the earth longer than any person alive today. The trees have seen things people today have not seen; they have felt the earth shake in ways the people of today have not felt. Because children have eyes to see what the adults cannot, the trees are not afraid to talk to them. If a child knows to seek out the wisdom of a tree, and has an open heart to believe it, the tree will bestow its wisdom upon the child. Children all over the world have approached the trees with their deepest struggles, and through their conversations have found how to make their daily lives better. The children can come to the tree with problems at home, hard feelings, or other challenges, and they will receive wisdom.

Such trees are called Wisdom Trees, and they can be found around the world. One such tree exists in the heart of New York City. Every child in the area knows of the Wisdom Tree, which stands in the west end of Central Park. When a child needs advice or someone to listen and express care for them, the Wisdom Tree is always there, waiting patiently. The Wisdom Tree is full of knowledge, from how to remain calm when things get hard, to being present and finding beauty at the moment, to learning how to treat others kindly and safely. The Wisdom Tree makes every child who visits feel safe, seen, and heard, and every child walks away with a lighter heart and a calmer mind. In this story, you will listen to three children who paid visits to the Wisdom Tree from all over New York.

***

Part 1: Cultivating Kindness

The first child to come to the tree was Jack. Although it was getting late, Jack could not wait any longer to speak to the Wisdom Tree. He had taken the subway from school that day to Central Park, where he had heard the Wisdom Tree resided. As he wandered through Central Park, searching for the signature large trunk and branches that hung like arms of a warm embrace, he wondered if the Wisdom Tree was indeed here as he had heard from the other children.

Suddenly, he stumbled across it. The large trunk was ridged like a wise face, with hanging branches that made Jack feel safe. The early evening sunlight glimmered gold through the branches like emeralds, and Jack knew from the feeling in his heart that he was at the right place. "Wisdom Tree?" he spoke hesitantly. "Hello," the omniscient voice echoed. It was peaceful and seemed to hang in the air between the two of them. "How can I help you today, child?"

"I've come here today because of something I saw at school. It's something I've seen for a while. But it was especially bad today," Jack began. The Wisdom Tree did not speak, instead held the space for Jack to continue. "There is a boy in my class named Gus. He wears thick, lime-green glasses that strap to the back of his head. He speaks more slowly than the other kids and has more trouble in class, and when individual lights or sounds bother him, he gets distraught.

The kids in my class, especially the group of boys who are friends with Kaden Duncan, like to make fun of him. Some kids don't make fun of him, but they're not his friends. No one in my class is friends with him. Sometimes, Kaden and the boys will laugh or make jokes when Gus tries to speak up in class or when he starts to get upset about something. They call him names. Sometimes when he's in the hallway, they'll push his body out of the way with their bodies. And sometimes, they punch him in the arm with the jokes they make. He doesn't like that."

"You've never stood of for Gus, is that right?" asked the Wisdom Tree. "No, I haven't," Jack replied sheepishly. "I don't know how to talk to him or what my classmates might think if I did." "I see," the Wisdom Tree responded.

"And Wisdom Tree, today was the worst day of all. See, Gus was sitting out by the sandbox on the playground. He likes to put the sand in his palm and look at it. Well, Kaden and the boys came up behind him and started calling him horrible names and kicking sand at his head. He started yelling and getting upset, and they just kept going, kicking the sand and making fun of him. When they were done, they pushed him, and he fell into the grass by the edge of the sandbox. After that, he just laid there for a while, until finally, he was able to pull himself up, and we went inside."

"Did anyone tell the teacher?" asked the Wisdom Tree. "I don't think so. Everyone is too afraid that we would become the next victims of Kaden and his boys if we did.

I am too afraid of people not liking me or thinking I'm weird. But I couldn't stop thinking about this all day long. I feel a sad feeling in my heart, and I don't know what to do about it." The Wisdom Tree sat in silence for a moment, thinking and letting the feelings of the moment sink in. "Jack, this story seems to me like a lesson in kindness, especially as it pertains to being a bystander in a situation of bullying. Do you know what a bystander is?" "No," Jack answered, "I haven't heard of that before."

"A bystander is what you and everyone else who saw what happened to Gus was today. You watched something dangerous and hurtful happening to another person, and you may have felt bad, but you didn't stand up for the person. Sometimes, people are bystanders because they're too afraid to stand up—afraid that they might get hurt themselves or that other people will not like them or make fun of them. Other people are bystanders because since the situation isn't happening to them, they can't make themselves care enough to do anything. They assume that someone else will take care of it, and they just walk away without letting it affect them. In our conversation, you have made it clear to me that you were a bystander because you were afraid, not because you didn't care."

"Yes," Jack said, "I guess that's right."

"The Wisdom I'm going to give you today is about kindness. From the time children are young, you are taught to be kind to others. So why do these things happen? It's because there are so many aspects of kindness that aren't talked about. Real kindness requires at least one of the following three things: unconditionality, compassion/Empathy, and courage. We will talk about what each of those means and how you can use them as tools to make you a kinder person in your own life.

***

"First, let's talk about conditionality," said the Wisdom Tree, "One thing about kindness that nobody tells you is that it is much easier to be kind on our terms. Although it shouldn't be, kindness is often conditional. Do you know what I mean when I say kindness is conditional?"

"Does it mean not everyone gets it?" asked Jack. "Sort of," the Wisdom Tree answered, "It means that we pick and choose who 'deserves' our kindness. It is much easier to be kind to the people that we already know and care about. It is much harder to be kind to a stranger because people don't often look at the strangers they pass on the street and think of the fact that they have a life just as complex as your own. It is even more challenging to be kind to people who are not kind to us back. People establish conditions around kindness by imagining that if someone is not kind to them, that person doesn't deserve to be treated well in return. The problem with the way many people think about kindness is that it doesn't always come from wanting to make the world better, but rather making our relationships better, being perceived as a good person, or receiving something in return. Even though kindness should be more about the other person than it is about you, that's not the way most people think about it."

Jack thought for a moment. His mind went to his mother, telling him to be kind to his teachers so that they would like him and be a good student. When his mother told him this, she wasn't telling him to be kind because his teachers were human beings that deserved kindness, but because they were human beings that could give him something if they liked him. "Yes," he responded, "I see what you mean. But Wisdom Tree, I have a question. If kindness isn't conditional, does that mean that kindness should go not only to Gus but also to his bullies?"

"Essentially, yes. It is essential to extend kindness to Gus, to protect him and be his friend, simply because all humans deserve compassion. But that doesn't mean that you would treat his bullies poorly by calling them names, shoving them in the hall, or kicking sand at their heads. You would not need to be friends with them, but they still need to be treated with human decency, even though they have been cruel. At the end of the day, all human beings need kindness. Sometimes, the power of service is enough to change the hearts of those who are especially unkind.

***

"Compassion and empathy are two things that people often think are similar, but in reality, they have many differences," the Wisdom Tree said. "Empathy is approaching a situation from a feeling perspective. When you can put yourself in someone else's shoes and feel the things they're feeling. Compassion is when, although you don't know how it feels to go through what a particular person is going through, you approach their situation with understanding and hold space to hear about their experience and show care for them within that."

"What if I can't make myself feel what someone else is feeling?" Jack asked, "What if I can't experience emotions that don't happen to me?" "You're not alone on that," the Wisdom Tree responded, "In fact, most people can't experience deep Empathy for everyone that they meet. It is challenging for most people to feel other people's feelings, especially people they don't know well or don't think fondly of. When it comes to kindness, compassion is very often more important than Empathy."

"How does a person practice compassion?" Jack asked. "Compassion is a choice you make every day when you wake up in the morning, and that you keep making throughout the day every time you forget," said the Wisdom Tree. "Tell me, Jack, what do you do when you get up in the morning?"

"I wake up, lay in bed for a few minutes, then get up, get dressed, brush my teeth, and eat Cheerios for breakfast," Jack answered, "After that, I walk down the street to the subway station and take the subway to school."

"So, when the sun first shines through your window in the morning, that is when compassion begins. In those moments, when you are lying in bed, preparing to get up, think about what compassion looks like. Take a few deep breaths, imagining your heart opening up to the stories of every person you meet. Imagine the feeling of telling them, 'I don't know what it feels like to be in your position, but I care about you, and I want to show you.' Then, keep coming back to the feeling of openness in your heart over and over again throughout the day. As you see people on the subway, in the halls at school, or in the grocery store, you can say a silent prayer in your head that says, 'No matter where you're at in your life; I want to extend peace and blessings to you.' This is an act of compassion in itself, even though no one can hear it out loud."

"That sounds great," said Jack, "but it also sounds hard to do." "It is hard to do," answered the Wisdom Tree, "and that's why it takes practice. See, there is a special part of the brain that shows compassion, and just like any muscle in the body, you have to work this part of the brain. The more you practice compassion and bring attention to it, the stronger this part of your brain becomes. As it becomes stronger, you won't have to think about it as much." "So, how can I bring this wisdom to the situation with Gus?" Jack asked. "Well, because you have never been pushed, or mocked, or had sand kicked at your head as Gus has, you cannot bring the understanding of someone who knows how that feels. But what you can do is imagine how it might feel, or even more importantly, approach Gus from a position of understanding that he must feel extremely hurt by how he has been treated. The best way to approach this situation would be to approach Gus and get to know him. Listen as he tells you about his struggles daily, about the pain and confusion and loneliness he feels. Then, once you understand his situation better, you can respond to him better as a friend."

"What if Gus doesn't want to be friends with me?" Jack asked. "That's okay, too," said the Wisdom Tree, "You can still show him compassion by standing up for him when other students make fun of or hurt him, not because you know the feeling, but because you understand how horrible it must feel. You can also show compassion by asking Gus what you can do to make him feel better and safer at school. Let him know that you see the difficulty in what he is going through, listen to what he says he needs, and let him know that you have his back."

Gus nodded. "Okay, I think I understand compassion a little more now. I have learned that I don't have to know exactly how it feels to be in someone else's shoes to care and want to do what I can to make other people's lives better. And I understand that this is something every person deserves."

***

"Wonderful," spoke the Wisdom Tree. "Now that we have addressed conditionality and the difference between compassion and Empathy, let's talk about courage. Earlier, you said you were too afraid to stand up for Gus or approach him to become his friend. Why are you afraid?"

"I'm afraid to stand up for him because what if the boys decide to start hurting me or laughing at me and making me feel embarrassed in front of the class? What if I lose friends, or people see me as weak?" Jack asked. "So you're afraid of the way people are going to see you, or maybe that they will start treating you the same way they treat Gus, is that right?" "Yes," Jack admitted. "I want you to think about something," said the Wisdom Tree. "If you saw another child run over to Gus this afternoon on the playground, would you have felt braver to join them?" "Yes," Jack said, "If I knew I wasn't going to be alone, I wouldn't have felt so afraid to help Gus." "So, if another person taking the first step to act kind could make you feel braver too, don't you think you could make another person feel that way?"

"Yes, I guess I could," said Jack. "The thing about kindness, Jack, is that it has the power to start a whole movement. But someone has to be brave enough to take the first step. If you take the first step to show kindness to Gus, your other classmates who want to help but are too afraid to speak up are likely to join in your movement. As the group of students who protect Gus and treat him with kindness grows, they will become stronger, and as this group becomes stronger, Kaden and his boys will become weaker. The more people who join the movement of kindness, the less power cruelty holds. And I will tell you this, Jack, kindness will always come out on top. Yes, you may have to risk being laughed at when you first begin. You may have to risk being called a name or even having sand kicked at your head. But when your classmates see that someone has stepped beyond the fear, they will be inspired to do the same. Soon enough, the bullies will not be able to hurt Gus anymore, nor will they have the power to hurt any of the rest of you. It is even possible that they may give in to the power of kindness themselves, apologizing to Gus, and becoming better people in the future. That is the power of kindness. Love has the power to overwhelm all fear," said the Wisdom Tree, "The question here, Jack, is are you brave enough to take the first step?"

"I don't know if I am brave enough," Jack admitted, "I still feel afraid." "It's okay to be afraid, Jack. What isn't okay is allowing that fear to control you. Come on now; we are going to do some meditations on kindness. These meditations will open your heart, melt away your fear, and help you come into a place of true kindness towards others."

***

"To begin, sit down in the grass with a straight back and close your eyes," instructed the Wisdom Tree. "Now, I want you to begin to breathe in and out, in and out. Breathe in love; breathe out fear. Bring your attention to your body. What sensations are there? Do you feel any tingling or tightness? Pay attention to the beating of your heart and the pace of your breath.

Are your breaths deep like an ocean or shallow like a tidepool? Are they quick or slow? No matter what you notice in your body, let it be there. Do not try to change anything."

"Now, I want you to bring your attention to your heart. Imagine a rose in a garden, sparkling in dewdrops in the morning. Imagine as the sun rises, the petals of the rose opening up to the sky to take in the day. Now, I want you to imagine your heart as the same thing—a rose opening at dawn. Imagine all people everywhere, having space in your heart. They are deserving of love simply because they exist. Imagine your heart filling up with kindness for each of them. Imagine the light coming out of your chest as you do kind things for other people.

Allow yourself to sit in the warmth of that open-hearted light. Keep breathing."

The two sat in silence for a few moments, breathing slowly. After a little while, the Wisdom Tree spoke again. "Now, we will practice melting away the fear. Bring your attention back to your body, and feel the place where fear gathers. What color is it? Does it feel heavy? Cold? Thick? Where does it come from?"

"Now, imagine the rays of the sun, shining down on the fear in your body and making it melt. As it melts away, imagine it turning into love. What color is love? Whatever color your love is, let the fear take that shape and begin to float freely through your body. Feel the lightness of being set free from your fear. Even when bad things happen, you can allow them to move through you simply, and you can maintain your courage through and through."

"Lastly, I want you to imagine yourself smiling and holding the people you meet in your heart. How will you bless the people around you with kindness today? I want you to send up a prayer that says, 'Please show me how to be kind today.' Imagine yourself having a clear enough head and an open enough heart to see the opportunities to be kind to others and take them whenever you get the chance. Remind yourself that you are kind not to receive anything in return, but rather because kindness is your purpose. Say this to yourself over and over again as you breathe. *My purpose is kindness. My purpose is kindness. My purpose is kindness.*"

As Jack did this, he felt his body become light and warm, and his heart opened wide. He felt more joy and peace than he had ever felt, and he knew that never again would he stand by and allow cruelty to take place. "My purpose is kindness," he said to himself. "Thank you, Wisdom Tree."

Part 2: Softening Anger

Her steps were determined but light as she walked through the cascading trees of Central Park. The leaves crushed beneath her as she continued on her path, nervous but hopeful. She stopped for a second and looked up at the sky, taking a deep breath and calming herself. As soon as she was centered, she heard a soft voice echoing through the trees: "Child, why are you so solemn?" She gasped and glanced around her, looking for the source of the words. She set her sights on a kind pair of eyes. She gulped and said, "He-hello. Are you the Wisdom Tree?" The eyes that were staring back at her softened, and the mouth smiled before saying, "Yes, that is me. Why are you here, young one? What troubles you?"

The girl sighed with relief and said, "I have a problem that I don't know how to fix." The Wisdom Tree invited her to sit and share, so the girl did. "What is your name?" said the tree, and the girl replied, "Charlotte. My name is Charlotte." The Wisdom Tree smiled and said, "Hello Charlotte, it is very nice to meet you. Would you like to share your troubles with me?" Charlotte nodded nervously, unsure of how to start. The tree's eyes softened again as she gave a reassuring smile, telling Charlotte, "It's okay. This is a safe space, and you can share anything you would like with me."

Charlotte nodded and began, "Well, I overheard my parents talking about me yesterday. They were angry and concerned. They said I had anger issues and that they didn't know what to do with me." The tree gave another comforting smile, "That is okay, child. Do you know why they said those things?"

Charlotte shook her head, yes, and the tree continued, "Do you have stories you would like to share?" Charlotte responded with, "Yes," but her voice was filled with nerves. She took a deep breath and started. "I have issues at school. My teacher is always telling me to calm down, but I don't know how. I get so angry." The tree understood, saying, "Everybody gets angry sometimes. Do you know why you get that way?" Charlotte shed a tear and said, "Yes, I think so. The other kids in class make fun of me sometimes. I just moved here, and they don't like new and strange things. I tried to make friends, but no one wanted to be friends with me. They didn't like the food I brought for lunch, they made fun of the clothes I wear, and I started yelling at them."

The tree replied, "Moving somewhere new can be very challenging. Some children can treat you differently because they don't understand you. Where did you move from, child?" More tears fell as Charlotte responded, "Chicago. My daddy got a new job here, and we had to move. I had to leave all my friends at my old school, and I don't know anybody here." The tree looked sad for a second as she said, "I am so sorry to hear that. This is a challenging time for you. It is okay to feel anger. How do you feel when the other children say mean things to you?" Charlotte wiped the tears off her cheeks and said, "It feels bad. At first, I was sad and lonely, and then I got furious at them. I would start yelling mean things back to them, and one Time I pushed a girl down at recess. I was so mad at her. She said I was weird and that my clothes looked old. My teacher yelled at me that day and called my parents. I got grounded, but that only made me angrier. The next day, I went to school and was mean to everyone, even the kids that have never said mean things to me. I don't know why I feel like this. I don't know how to stop it."

The tree sighed and responded, "Child, these feelings are natural. It is okay to feel sad and angry, but acting on these feelings only makes other people feel sad. How do you think the other kids felt when you said mean things to them, but they had never said those things to you? Charlotte started crying more, and she sniffed as she said, "Bad. I think they felt the same way I felt. I don't know how to stop. I was so angry at the other kids that I just, well, I don't know." Charlotte stuttered and didn't know what else to say. The tree smiled and responded, "Making other kids feel the way you did won't fix your anger. Your anger is only your own, and the only way to heal from that anger is to forgive."

Charlotte gasped, "Forgive? How could I forgive what those other kids said to me? They hurt me!" The tree replied, "Forgiveness will not come easily. Forgiveness is difficult, and it takes time. Do you want to stop feeling angry?" Charlotte nodded. The tree continued, "The mean things those kids said to you are not okay, but their anger is only coming from another place in them, just as your anger to the kids who did nothing to you came from the mean things you heard. Do you understand?" Charlotte nodded slightly with a confused look, "So, the mean kids are only mean because someone was mean to them?" The tree replied, "Sometimes, yes. We all get angry, and sometimes we take our anger out on the people who did nothing to deserve it. Many people don't know how to control our strong feelings, so we take out our aggression on someone else. You responded to the mean comments by taking your anger out on everyone else. Have you ever been mad at your parents and said bad things to them when they didn't deserve it?" Charlotte nodded, "Yes. I would come home from school and lock myself in my room. They would try to talk to me and comfort me, but I wouldn't listen. I only yelled at them to go away. One Time I even said I hated them," Charlotte started crying again but continued, "I don't hate my parents. I don't know why I said that." The tree looked at Charlotte and said, "You said those things because you didn't know how to deal with your anger. You were doing the same thing those mean kids were doing to you.

***

"I will tell you what," the Wisdom Tree spoke, "let's talk about new ways to deal with your anger when it arises. There are many ways to address your anger without letting it take control of you; sometimes, we just need to be aware of the tools that exist in our toolbox and have them ready to use when we need them."

"First of all, let's determine where anger lives in your body. If it had a hiding place, where would it be?" "I think my anger sits in my stomach," Charlotte said, "but when it begins to get worse, it rises through my throat and makes my face feel hot and scrunchy. I feel m body tighten up, and sometimes I feel it explode out of me. Sometimes it explodes like fire through my fingers and makes me want to hit or throw. Other times, it explodes through my mouth, and my voice gets loud."

"You may not feel like it's okay to have these explosive feelings, but it is," the Wisdom Tree said,

"When we have feelings, they need somewhere to go. But you already know that if your anger, I think we should make a safe landing place for your anger comes out in a way that hurts somebody else, that isn't good. Why don't we try to make a safe place for your body to let your anger out? A place where no one will get hurt?"

"Like where?" Charlotte asked. She was confused because she had never heard of anger as something that deserved to be let out. She also couldn't think of anger as being let out safely. "What if you made a landing place for your anger?" the Wisdom Tree asked, "somewhere with thick, soft things like blankets or pillows. These are safe things that can take all the force of your yelling, angry words, and angry hand movements without making anyone else get hurt. When the anger is exploding out your mouth, you can scream into a pillow as long and as loud as you want. This keeps the anger from getting stuck inside you, but it also keeps it from hitting and hurting anyone else. Words can't be erased after they have been said, and screams can be scary, so you can keep the people in your life safe by having a place to yell into. And when the anger explodes out your fingers, you can use the pillow for that too. You can wind up your body like a slinky, letting all your energy wind up, then letting it go into a big hit onto the soft-landing spot of the pillow. You can keep hitting it, letting all your energy come out again and again until there is none of it left in your body."

"What do I do after all my angry energy is out of my body?" Charlotte asked, "What if I don't feel ready to go back to the world yet?" "You can stay in your own special space until you feel calm. Sometimes, it's good to make a quiet corner for yourself with all your blankets, pillows, and other soft-landing places for your emotions. You can keep coloring books, stuffed animals, or journals there to help you calm down afterward and get yourself back into a place where you can be calm and have fun again," the Wisdom Tree advised.

"Another way to deal with your anger is to get to know it. Ask your anger what it is doing there. Is it trying to teach you something? Maybe there is another feeling, like embarrassment, shame, sadness, or loneliness that is taking up a lot of space in your body, and the anger feels like it has to take action to make it better. Whatever is making you angry, there is always more of a reason. If you become angry at the kids on the playground calling you names and want to hit them or call them names back, where do you think that anger might be coming from?" the Wisdom Tree asked.

Charlotte thought for a moment. "I guess it comes from feeling sad when people call me names. I just want the people at school to be friends with me, ask me questions, and not think that I'm weird. I don't want to be lonely or have people make fun of me," she said. "Exactly," responded the Wisdom Tree, "so in that case, your anger is coming from a place of hurt in being called names, loneliness in feeling ignored by the other kids, and perhaps confused as to why they are treating you this way. All of those feelings make a lot of sense. Our bodies don't hold feelings for no reason—there is always a reason for the feelings we have, and we have to have the courage to ask them what they want us to know."

"Wisdom Tree, how do I know where my anger comes from, and how to understand it better?"

Charlotte asked. "You can make a list every single day of the things that made you feel angry on a certain day, then ask yourself what other feelings made that anger come. Were you sad or embarrassed? Did you feel ignored? Knowing why your anger comes is the most important way to honor it, without letting it hurt you or the people around you," the Wisdom Tree said.

"Wisdom Tree," Charlotte spoke again, "I understand that everybody gets angry and that I shouldn't get angry at my anger. But it's so hard when I can't even understand the things that make me feel angry before they do. How can I keep myself from exploding before it's too late?" "You ask a good question, child," responded the Wisdom Tree, "A good way to do this is to make a list of the things that made you feel the fire in you rising most easily. Do you feel it when people aren't listening to you? When you're told 'no'? When you lose a game? When you get stuck and can't figure something out?

When people tease you? When you're hungry, thirsty, or tired? When you feel rushed? When someone takes something away from you? When someone hurts your body? Knowing the things that make the fire of anger start to rise in, you can help you be prepared to get it under control before it starts burning you and the people around you."

"I think the things that make me most angry are being called names and when I feel like people aren't listening to me. I want to feel like people value what I have to say, and as they respect me enough not to tease me," Charlotte said.

The Wisdom Tree sat patiently for a few moments to let the silence sink in before continuing. "Charlotte, I want you to imagine if your anger was a person. What kind of person would it be?" Charlotte scratched her head in thought. "I think my anger would be the kind of person who walks with hunched shoulders, ready to spring forward like a slinky at any time. They would have a big red face with hair like flames, and their eyes would be black. My anger would be loud and move around in difficult ways, and it might make other people feel afraid. Almost like a monster, except it isn't a monster; it just needs some water and deep breaths to calm down."

"Now," said the Wisdom Tree, "let's try to imagine ways that you can stop your anger from getting out of hand once you start to feel that it is there. When you get angry, your nervous system starts to get fiery and bunched up. Luckily, there is an extraordinary secret for coming back into the moment and helping your nervous system unwind. That secret is breathing." "Breathing?" Charlotte asked, "How can that be a secret when we do it all day, every day?" The Wisdom Tree seemed to smile. "Most people don't realize this, but because your breathing happens without you having to do anything, it can bring you back down to earth when you feel out of control and help you to find a sense of peace and safety. There are a few ways that you can use your breathing to help your anger cool down. Let's try them together."

"First of all, I want you to take all ten of your fingers and put them up in front of you," the Wisdom Tree directed. Charlotte did as she was asked. "Now, I want you to pretend these are the candles on a birthday cake. You blow out the candles on your birthday cakes, don't you?" the Wisdom Tree asked. "Yes, I do," Charlotte answered. "Good.

So, imagine each of these fingers is a candle and blow it out as slowly as possible. Blow until you feel all the air in your tummy go out into the world.

As you blow, imagine all the sad and dangerous energy inside you unraveling and flowing out into the world to be recycled into something healthier, just like plants recycle carbon dioxide. Keep blowing out each candle slowly, one by one, letting everything boiling inside of you come out."

"Next, let's imagine we're going to breathe to make a rainbow. Have you ever seen a rainbow, Charlotte?" the Wisdom Tree asked. "Yes, I love rainbows!" Charlotte exclaimed. "Rainbows come after storms. The storm may be scary, but the rain makes it so new things can grow on the earth. Rainbows stretch across the sky that change is good sometimes, and sometimes, the only way growth can happen is after a storm. Let's practice making a rainbow with our breath, and each time you breathe in, I want you to imagine something new growing in the places inside you where the anger once was," the Wisdom Tree instructed.

Together, the two began breathing in, and Charlotte imagined the bottom of an arch. She breathed in, imaging making the half-arc of a rainbow. "You can do any color you like until you feel your rainbow is complete," the Wisdom Tree said. Slowly, Charlotte breathed in, drawing arches of every color, especially purples and blues, until the rainbow looked precisely the way she wanted, and she felt calm inside.

"Okay," spoke the Wisdom Tree, "we are going to try one more type of special breathing to calm anger now. Have you ever made a wish on a dandelion?" "Yes," Charlotte spoke, "I love making wishes on dandelions and watching the seeds fly far and wide like small fairies scattered to the wind." "We are going to scatter wishes to the wind with this breathing style, too," said the Wisdom Tree, "as you breathe in, I want you to imagine breathing in good things. Breathe in joy, breathe in calm, breathe in strength. As you breathe out, imagine that you are blowing on a dandelion, spreading good things far and wide to the earth. Breathe out and make a wish. Say 'I wish to be kind to others.' 'I wish to keep the calm inside of me.' 'I wish to help others in any way I can.' 'I wish to learn what I can from the things that happen to me.' As you breathe out, imagine each of the seeds taking root in the earth and blooming into something brand new and beautiful."

***

When Charlotte opened her eyes, the Wisdom Tree was still there, waiting patiently for her to come back. "How do you feel?" the Wisdom Tree asked her. "I feel like I do when I fall asleep next to my mom, or when I am lying in the sand by the ocean or lying in a field of flowers. I feel less afraid of my anger. I feel kinder and stronger, and like I understand myself for once. I know now that I do not have to force my anger away with more anger, but instead, I can treat it like an old friend who can teach me and from whom I can make new and beautiful things grow. Thank you, Wisdom tree."

Part 3: Calming Anxiety

The third child to come to the tree was called Evalyn. Evalyn was too afraid to go to Central Park alone, so when her family came to Central Park for a picnic, she stole away for a few moments, saying she wanted to go for a walk. Evalyn walked along, looking this way and that for the distinguished Wisdom Tree she had heard so much about. Recently, Evalyn had been to so many doctors, but none of them quite seemed to help her.

Finally, she saw it, the legendary tree with the ridges that seemed to make a face and the branches that hung low and full of love.

Looking at the tree, Evalyn immediately felt some of the rushings in her heart slow down, and some of the buzzing in her head begin to quiet. She walked up to the Wisdom Tree and felt her voice catch in her throat. She was too scared to say hello. Luckily, Wisdom Tree spoke up first. "Hello, Evalyn," spoke the echoing voice that immediately made Evalyn's soul feel as calm as a pond with no ripples. "What can I help you with today?"

"Wisdom Tree," Evalyn stammered, "I feel like my head is a buzzing beehive. The thoughts and fears come in and out and in and out, and I just can't even think straight.

My mother keeps taking me to the doctor because we don't know why I can't sleep at night or why every Time I get dropped off at dance class, I become afraid my mother won't come back. When we have to do our spelling tests in school, my brain convinces me that every word is wrong, even when I spend hours studying. Sometimes when it happens, my breathing gets so fast that I have to leave the room and go to the bathroom. I sit on the toilet with my head in my hands and feel like I'm dying because I can't catch my breath. Sometimes an adult has to come in and help me. Once, I threw up and was so anxious I couldn't talk, and my mom had to come to get me from school. I am so afraid of chemicals getting in my mouth that sometimes I spit on the ground just to be sure. I can't fall asleep at night because I feel scared that I won't wake up the next day. I get so frightened about a fire coming to my house. When I try to speak in class, even when I know the answer, my brain tells me I don't know, and I feel my vocal cords tying themselves in knots and lose my voice. This is the only time my mind becomes quiet—when I forget what it was, I needed to say, and the entire world becomes black."

Evalyn was speaking so fast, and her breathing was hard and quick. The Wisdom Tree said gently, with a calm and even tone. "So, you feel like every thought and worry is a bee, buzzing around in the hive that is your brain, right?" "Right," said Evalyn, "That's exactly how I feel. And the buzzing sound makes it so hard to relax and have fun or focus on anything I need to do. All I can think of is the fact that I can never find quiet. We go to the doctor to try to find a way to make my brain quiet again, but nothing seems to work. I am afraid of everything; even when there is nothing to be afraid of, I always find something. I just can't help it."

***

"It is so scary to feel like you are always in a fight with your brain," said the Wisdom Tree, "and it is so hard to be distracted by the things our brains tell us constantly. When you have anxiety, that means that your brain is more likely to tell you to be afraid of things or worry about things that will not happen. The good news is, there are so many ways to gain control again—to tell your brain, 'I'm not going to let you tell me this.' Let's talk about them."

"First of all, what are the things that make the bees in your beehive brain buzz fastest?" The Wisdom Tree asked, "What are you most afraid of?" "I'm terrified of being alone. My brain always tells me that my mom will leave me when I get dropped off somewhere like a school or a dance class. I'm also terrified of speaking in class.

My brain always tells me that I don't know what I'm talking about, that I'm going to give the wrong answer, and that my classmates will laugh at me."

"Okay," said the Wisdom Tree, "The first way to get these fears to calm down is to let them be there. Let's think of a real bee, for example. If a bee flies up to you, do you start yelling and swatting it away in fear, or do you allow it to be there and fly around for a bit until the moment passes and the bee goes on its way?" "You're not supposed to yell or swat it, or it might become afraid and sting you," Evalyn answered. "Exactly," said the Wisdom Tree, "think of your biggest anxiety thoughts like this. When something comes up in your brain that makes you feel afraid, let it be there. Say to yourself, 'I know this is my brain telling me that I don't know what I'm talking about. It's okay to be afraid; I'm going to let that fear be here and then drift away just as soon as it came.' Take some time to breathe into that space, imagining that fear flying around for a little bit, then going back the same direction it came. We can't face our fears unless we recognize what they are."

"Another place where anxiety comes from is feeling like we have to be perfect. When you raise your hand in class, your brain tells you that you have to get everything right or you're not smart. This isn't true at all. As humans, we are all imperfect. We all make mistakes, and that is often how we learn the best. It's okay if you answer a question wrong in class or do the wrong step at your dance recital. Instead of looking at the fear of not being perfect, ask yourself, what do you love about things like school and dance?"

"At school, I love to write stories. It's so much fun to design the characters and decide what happens to them and what choices they make. And at dance class, I love to learn new combinations. It is so fun to make my body move to music—I especially like doing pirouette turns," Evalyn responded. "Great!" spoke the Wisdom Tree, "so now, when you go to school, or dance class, or anywhere else, I want you to remind yourself why you are there. You are at school to learn, and one of the things you love learning most is how to write stories. You are at dance class to move your body and make art to music, and one of the things you love most is doing pirouettes. Let your school be about learning and writing stories, and your dance be about movement and feeling free as you do your pirouettes. It isn't about how well you do it; it is about how much you enjoy it. If you have learned something and it has made you smile, that is all the success you could ever ask for."

***

"Let me ask you another thing," the Wisdom Tree said, "What makes you feel relaxed?" Evalyn thought for a moment. "I feel calm when I listen to piano music," she said, "and when I sit in the garden in the mornings or look at the stars at night."

"Those are things you need to make time for every day," said the Wisdom Tree, "Whenever you feel anxious, give yourself time just to sit. Look at the nature around you, or put on piano music. Do whatever you need to do to bring yourself back down. Every day as you plan out what you will do, make sure to schedule a time to relax. Let yourself play, and just have fun."

"What about when I'm in a moment, and my beehive brain starts buzzing too much, and I lose control?" asked Evalyn, "What do I do then?" "I am so happy you asked," said the Wisdom Tree, "I have a trick for that." "The best way to bring yourself back to earth when your brain starts to take you somewhere else is by paying attention to the senses. What do you hear? What do you see? What do you smell? What do you feel? When you feel yourself start to panic, find a place to step away, and start to look around you. Find something you can see. After you have found that, breathe that thing in until you begin to see again, and the darkness fades away. Then, find something you can hear. What are the sounds around you? Find one to focus on. After that, find something you can feel. Can you reach out and touch an object nearby, or feel the wind or sun on your skin? What about smell or taste? Let's try this exercise right now so you can practice."

"Okay," said Evalyn. "So," spoke the Wisdom Tree, "what's something you can see right now?" Evalyn looked around them. "I see a robin on the ground; it looks like he's digging for worms." "Good," said the Wisdom Tree, "now pay special attention to that robin and breathe as you do it. That robin is a sign that you are here, this is real, and you are okay. You and this robin are here together, and you are both okay." "Next, let's find something you can hear. Pay attention to the sounds around us and let me know what sticks with you," the Wisdom Tree said. Evalyn listened carefully. There were many sounds in the park, but the one she found herself most drawn to was the sound of a group of teenagers playing soccer nearby. "I hear people having a fun game of soccer. I hear them laughing, talking to each other, and the sound of their feet on the ball when they kick it."

"Great," said the Wisdom Tree, "let yourself sit for a few moments, breathing into that sound. Remind yourself that this is real, and you are all here together." "Wow, this does make me feel calmer," said Evalyn. "Now, let's try another," said the Wisdom Tree, "Pay attention to something that you can feel." Evalyn closed her eyes and paid attention to her body. "I feel the breeze. It's not too hot or too cold; the air feels just right. It makes me feel good," she said. "Now, allow yourself to stay here, feeling this sensation in your body," said the Wisdom Tree, "Breathe with it and let it remind you that you are here and you are safe." After a few moments passed, the Wisdom Tree spoke again, "Time for us to go into a new sensation. Here, we will see if there is anything you can smell or taste. These things are not always as easy, but they can help to ground you too." "I smell the hotdogs from the stand nearby," said Evalyn "they smell smoky and delicious." "Good," spoke the Wisdom Tree, "now if it helps, imagine eating them, or think about what the smell of hotdogs reminds you of." "It reminds me of being in my uncle's backyard for a barbecue," Evalyn said.

"And that is a place where you feel safe, right?" asked the Wisdom Tree. "Yes," Evalyn answered, "I feel very safe there because it is a place where I am having fun with my family." The two sat in this feeling of safety for a moment. "Now that you have learned how to bring yourself back into the world, it will be harder for your brain to keep you in a state of fear outside of your body," the Wisdom Tree said.

***

"Now, Evalyn," the Wisdom Tree spoke, "you have learned how to bring yourself back down if you start to become lost in your beehive brain. Let's talk about some ways that you can start your day with calm. When it comes to anxiety, you need to be friendly with it instead of being afraid. Facing your anxiety with friendliness and calm is something you have to do every morning to keep your brain in a healthy place. I'm going to teach you ten affirmations that can help you. With each one we do, I want you to imagine your beehive brain healing. I want you to imagine the golden sweetness of honey flowing out on everything you do."

"To start, you'll need to find a comfortable seat with a straight back. Close your eyes and let yourself come into the moment with deep breaths in and out. As you breathe in, say to yourself, 'I am breathing in all things well.' Feel your body expand as you breathe in good, happy, and calm things. When you breathe out, say to yourself, 'I am breathing out all things bad.' Let the fear, tension, and nervousness flow out of your body with the exhale. Imagine them as chains around your heart, loosening, and floating away."

Evalyn saw the image of the chains falling away and felt strong with every good thing she breathed in. "Now, I want you to imagine a pair of arms wrapping around you like a safe embrace. Settle into that feeling, and say to yourself, 'I am safe. I am safe. I am safe. That is affirmation number two," said the Wisdom Tree. As Evalyn did this, she felt her body relax as if she were once again a baby being held in her mother's arms. The tension in her body softened, and she did not feel afraid anymore.

"For affirmation number three, I want you to bring space to the parts of your body and brain where you feel anxiety. Acknowledge that it is there, and do not judge it or become angry with it. Breathe in and say to yourself, 'I am not my anxiety. I am not my anxiety. I am not my anxiety.' As you do this, feel those places in your body and brain soften into a golden light. Your anxiety is a part of you, but it is not who you are.

You are so much more," the Wisdom Tree said. At this point, Evalyn began to feel a soft yellow light, warming her entire body. "Now, we are going to talk about all of the things you are that your anxiety may try to make you feel that you are not.

Affirmation number four is this: 'I am strong. I am strong. I am strong.' As you say this, imagine yourself being able to handle any situation that comes your way with a sense of calm strength, knowing that you are capable of getting through anything and coming out on the other side. There is nothing to be afraid of," said the Wisdom Tree.

"Affirmation number five also has to do with strength," the Wisdom Tree said. Pay attention again to that place in your body or brain where your anxiety sits. Acknowledge that it is there, but then play into the acknowledgment that your strength is also there. Keep breathing and say to yourself, 'I have the strength to move beyond my anxiety. I have the strength to move beyond my anxiety. I have the strength to move beyond my anxiety.' Imagine yourself being set free, being able to enter a space where your anxiety does not have power over you."

"Affirmation number six is this: 'I look forward to a bright and happy future. I look forward to a bright and happy future. I look forward to a bright and happy future.' Although anxiety has made your world dark in the past, it does not have to be that way. There is a light in you that shines when you allow your anxiety to release its hold on you, and that light will pave the way into a beautiful and bright life. You can feel real joy in your life, and it will come." As she thought this, Evalyn's smile spread even wider across her face.

"Let's move to affirmation number seven. This is a visualization affirmation," the Wisdom Tree said. "I want you to bring your attention to that place in your belly at the center of your being. Imagine a pool of clear, sparkling water, with no ripples or waves, and nothing dirty or dangerous. Imagine a pool that is still, calm, and undisturbed. Even if something comes along to cause ripples or waves, which it always will, the pool returns to a state of calm reflection once the ripples pass. It holds onto its calm while the waves roll through, and eventually, they disappear, and a new moment comes. Be like this pond, saying to yourself, 'I give in to inner calm. I give in to inner calm. I give in to inner calm." Evalyn felt a whoosh of peace spreading throughout her middle. It was cold and refreshing, just like a crystal-clear pond.

"Now," spoke the Wisdom Tree, "As we move into affirmation number eight, I want you to imagine the days of your life. You already know that a 'perfect day' does not exist. Mistakes will be made, and things will not go as planned, and that's okay. When you speak up in class, perform on stage, or try something new, you cannot expect that it will always be just the way you want. But there is a comfort to be found in knowing that you are doing your best, and that is enough.

Affirmation number nine is just that: "I am doing my best, and that is enough. I am doing my best, and that is enough, I am doing my best, and that is enough."

"As we move into affirmation number nine, I want you to stay with the thought of things not always going as planned. You know that things will happen in life, causing ripples in your pond, and may cause the bees in your brain to buzz faster and louder. That is okay. The important thing is how you bring yourself back into space where you can keep moving forward. Affirmation number nine is a reminder to yourself that everything has a way of working itself out. 'I am going to be okay. I am going to be okay. I am going to be okay.' Say this to yourself as many times as it takes to believe it," said the Wisdom Tree. Evalyn began to try the method of telling herself she would be okay at that moment. She said it over and over again until she began to feel the truth of it within her, like a comforting hand stroking her hair and reassuring her.

"Last but not least," the Wisdom Tree spoke, "Affirmation number ten focuses on the power in the present moment to relieve you from anxiety. When people feel anxious, they feel anxious about things that they are afraid may happen in the future or things that have already happened in the past that cannot be changed. These fears are rooted in the helplessness that lies in a moment that is not the current one. By grounding yourself in the present moment, you will be able to experience a deeper sense of peace with what is happening around you and see your life for what it is without clouding it with the fears of what it once might happen in the future. Affirmation number ten is this: 'I allow myself to come into the present moment. I allow myself to come into the present moment. I allow myself to come into the present moment.' Evalyn, everything you need is available to you right here, right now. You just have to allow yourself to experience it."

Evalyn kept her eyes closed for a few moments longer. Her breathing had slowed and deepened, and she felt a blissful sense of calm spreading throughout her body. When she opened them again, the world looked clearer. There was not so much noise in her head, and she felt her heart had slowed to a healthy rate. She felt strength in her arms and legs and peace in the middle of her body that she had never felt. She was not afraid of what the next moment would bring because even if she got anxious, she had the tools within her to come back to a state of calm. The Wisdom Tree had taught her to live in peace with her beehive brain and find the strength in herself and the power in the present moment, to calm it down. She felt light shining out of her, and she knew her life was changed forever. "Thank you, wisdom tree," she said.

Conclusion:

Throughout this book, you and your child got to travel to fairy villages, faraway kingdoms, other cultures, wildflower gardens, and the most magical area of Central Park. You met children from all over the world, dealing with all kinds of things and receiving magical blessings, wisdom, guidance, and perspective. You saw fairies blessing children of the world with gratitude, understanding, body positivity, and relief from grief and sadness. You saw a horse who came on the full moon and took a little girl to multiple corners of the world so she could understand it better and learn how to communicate with people who come from other areas of the world, as well as figuring out what all people have in common. You saw princes who overcome the things they have always been told to do to treat the people of their kingdom with as much kindness as possible, make sure everyone has what they need, and learn lessons from humble places like gardens and the village below. You saw a Wisdom Tree that speaks to children from all over New York who learn how to be kind, protect other people, manage their anger, understand their feelings, and calm anxiety. All of these stories offered a new way for your child to engage their imagination, think about the world differently, and cultivate a sense of peace within themselves. Each story has been written to make your child feel seen, safe, and understood and extend that same understanding to other children they meet.

Overall, this book has provided several engaging stories to activate your children's imaginations and help them lean into the magical parts of life and being human. They have learned to open their minds and ask important questions when they need guidance. They have learned that it is okay to go through hard things and that there are many ways to grow from hard things. Lastly, these stories' calm tone helped your children rest peacefully and wake up feeling refreshed and ready to take on the world with all the tools they need for a happy and healthy life. Thank you for embarking on this journey.

Description

One incredible thing about a child's mind is easy access to the world beyond. Within the pages of this book, your child will embark on a magical journey through the concepts of open-mindedness, mindfulness, and emotional intelligence, through engaging stories of magic, exploration, and transcending expectations.

This book begins with stories about fairies living all over the world, cultivating their gifts and bringing blessings to children in all backgrounds and life situations. The fairies teach the children the power of gratitude, healing from grief, grounding in the present moment, appreciating the body they are in, learning self-love and self-acceptance, and finding the beauty in themselves and others. In the following story, you will read about how one girl's life changes from ordinary to extraordinary as she uncovers the secrets of other corners of the world on visits to India, the Amazon Rainforest, and a neighborhood of a city just like hers. She makes all of these visits during the three nights of the full moon on the back of a mystical moon horse who descends from the sky to teach her the greatest lessons of life. In the third story, you will explore a young prince's unlikely friendship with the kingdom gardener, and what he learns about compassion for others, and the strength that lies in being gentle. Over the course of the story, the prince finds his own voice, and musters up the strength to speak up for what he believes is right for all the people of his kingdom. In the final story, you will read the stories of the children who come to the Central Park Wisdom Tree for advice. The children explore the power of kindness, how to stand up to bullying, how to manage anger, calm anxiety, and find beauty in the way they learn.

Each of these stories is full of beautiful life lessons which will inform your child's thinking and help them to become more open, kind, and compassionate human beings. The soft, peaceful tone of the stories is perfect for bedtime and is sure to help your child wind down from the day and bring them to a night of blissful and restful sleep. When they fall asleep on the notes expressed in these stories, they will awaken feeling refreshed and ready to take on the world as the best versions of themselves they can possibly be. Additionally, the book gives you the opportunity to learn alongside your child, perhaps thinking of new perspectives you had not given much attention to in the past and learning how to integrate such topics into your child's life through the power of imagination and storytelling.

This book is designed to play into children's natural creativity, compassion, and curiosity to teach them stories combining fairytale creatures and other children worldwide. As you embark on this journey with your child, you will feel the power of a compassionate story, and together, you and your child can dive into your imaginations to make the world a better place.

www.ingramcontent.com/pod-product-compliance
Lightning Source LLC
Chambersburg PA
CBHW071618080526
44588CB00010B/1176